THE ARCHAEOLOGY OF AMERICAN MEDICINE AND HEALTHCARE

The American Experience in Archaeological Perspective

UNIVERSITY PRESS OF FLORIDA

Florida A&M University, Tallahassee
Florida Atlantic University, Boca Raton
Florida Gulf Coast University, Ft. Myers
Florida International University, Miami
Florida State University, Tallahassee
New College of Florida, Sarasota
University of Central Florida, Orlando
University of Florida, Gainesville
University of North Florida, Jacksonville
University of South Florida, Tampa
University of West Florida, Pensacola

The Archaeology of American Medicine and Healthcare

Meredith Reifschneider

Foreword by
Michael S. Nassaney and Krysta Ryzewski

UNIVERSITY PRESS OF FLORIDA

Gainesville/Tallahassee/Tampa/Boca Raton
Pensacola/Orlando/Miami/Jacksonville/Ft. Myers/Sarasota

This book will be made open access within three years of publication thanks to Path to Open, a program developed in partnership between JSTOR, the American Council of Learned Societies (ACLS), University of Michigan Press, and The University of North Carolina Press to bring about equitable access and impact for the entire scholarly community, including authors, researchers, libraries, and university presses around the world. Learn more at https://about.jstor.org/path-to-open/

Cover: Image from *American Medical Botany, Volume II*. Wikimedia Commons.

Copyright 2025 by Meredith Reifschneider
All rights reserved
Published in the United States of America

30 29 28 27 26 25   6 5 4 3 2 1

Library of Congress Cataloging-in-Publication Data
Names: Reifschneider, Meredith, author. | Nassaney, Michael S., author of
 foreword. | Ryzewski, Krysta, author of foreword.
Title: The archaeology of American medicine and healthcare / Meredith
 Reifschneider ; foreword by Michael S. Nassaney and Krysta Ryzewski.
Description: 1. | Gainesville : University Press of Florida, 2025. |
 Series: The American experience in archaeological perspective | Includes
 bibliographical references and index.
Identifiers: LCCN 2024025332 (print) | LCCN 2024025333 (ebook) | ISBN
 9780813079257 (hardback) | ISBN 9780813070872 (pdf) | ISBN 9780813073521
 (ebook)
Subjects: LCSH: Medical care—United States—History. | Medicine—United
 States—History. | Public health—United States—History. | BISAC:
 SOCIAL SCIENCE / Archaeology | MEDICAL / History
Classification: LCC R151 .R428 2025 (print) | LCC R151 (ebook) | DDC
 362.10973—dc23/eng/20241101
LC record available at https://lccn.loc.gov/2024025332
LC ebook record available at https://lccn.loc.gov/2024025333

The University Press of Florida is the scholarly publishing agency for the State University System of Florida, comprising Florida A&M University, Florida Atlantic University, Florida Gulf Coast University, Florida International University, Florida State University, New College of Florida, University of Central Florida, University of Florida, University of North Florida, University of South Florida, and University of West Florida.

University Press of Florida
2046 NE Waldo Road
Suite 2100
Gainesville, FL 32609
http://upress.ufl.edu

For my father, James Reifschneider, MD,
for your professional service, care, and unremitting compassion.

CONTENTS

List of Illustrations   ix
Foreword   xi
Acknowledgments   xix

1. Introduction   1
2. Professional Medicine and Archaeologies of the American Healthcare System   13
3. Healthcare Consumerism and Medicalization   46
4. Archaeologies of Public Health   74
5. Biocitizenship and Healthcare at the Presidio of San Francisco: The Moral Imperative of Health and Hygiene   113
6. Conclusion   144

References   159
Index   195

ILLUSTRATIONS

Figures

2.1. James Gillray, *Breathing a Vein* 17

2.2. Laënnec-type stethoscope 19

2.3. Estate Cane Garden hospital building, facing south 38

3.1. Lithograph advertisement for Hamlin's Wizard Oil 52

3.2. Lydia Pinkham's Vegetable Compound trade card 62

4.1. Five Points, New York, 1859 93

4.2. *The Salutation of Beatrice* (1869) 103

5.1. *Will You Be a Free Man or Chained?* 120

5.2. Victor Adam after Louis Choris, *Vue du Presidio san Francisco* 124

5.3. Presidio Building 104, now the Walt Disney Museum 127

5.4. Colgate Ribbon Dental Cream box from Building 104 130

5.5. Knoxit Injection bottle from Building 104 133

5.6. Larkspur Lotion bottle from Building 104 133

Table

5.1. Artifacts from Building 104 131

FOREWORD

Access to affordable and equitable healthcare, a long-term concern for most Americans, has come into sharper focus in the recent past during the political struggles over Obamacare and abortion. It became particularly salient during the COVID-19 global pandemic, which exposed the inability of our nationwide medical system to coordinate efficient responses to emergency care and vaccination. Perhaps for the first time in our lifetimes, no one felt safe; everyone faced the threat of contracting a deadly contagious disease. Americans were justifiably frightened in the early summer of 2020 as over 1,000 people were dying from COVID-19 each day. Quarantines were mandated, the vectors of transmission remained a mystery, and much of the population relied on essential workers to risk their lives in order to care for the sick and stock grocery shelves for basic necessities. Of course, the consequences of the pandemic fell disproportionately on those who were already medically, socially, and economically compromised, heightening their concerns and aggravating their burdens as they tried to stay healthy.

Material traces of our coping mechanisms were readily visible in the variety of face masks that were produced domestically and commercially. Toilet paper and cleaning supplies disappeared from the shelves of supermarkets. Grocers placed limits on nonperishable staples, like rice and flour, to prevent shoppers from hoarding necessities. Teddy bears displayed in windows and sidewalk chalk messages were designed to distract attention and buoy spirits among young and old alike. Not since the Great Depression did such desperation and uncertainty loom on the horizon. Our most hallowed medical institutions (hospitals, medical staff, the Centers for Disease Control and Prevention) offered seemingly conflicting advice regarding prevention and treatment, prompting a host of home remedies, ranging from ingesting Clorox bleach to sanitizing all surfaces thought to transmit the virus. Responses to COVID-19 were shaped by the distrust surrounding the uneven American experience of healthcare and medicine.

Many of us also look back at the early 2020s in mournful remembrance; few of us were spared friends, family, or associates who succumbed to the disease, and even years later this persistent virus regularly disrupts the best-laid plans for routine travel, celebrations, and large group events. We can only imagine how many more would have died in the United States and around the world had medical researchers failed to come to understand the virus's etiology, develop effective vaccines to keep it in check, and convince a small but critical segment of the population to follow protocols.

One would be hard-pressed to deny the efficacy of the role of medicine and healthcare in the American experience. Yet the pandemic laid bare the fact that not all Americans subscribe to scientific prescriptions for a host of reasons too numerous to detail. In *The Archaeology of American Medicine and Healthcare,* Meredith Reifschneider positions us to understand attitudes toward modern healthcare by looking backward to examine how Americans have coped with the processes of identifying and treating illness and disease. Because the outcomes of procedures as private as enemas, eye drops, and endoscopy are not widely shared, there is considerable uncertainty about their effectiveness and availability to various segments of the population. For historical reasons related to socioeconomic, racial, and gender bias, not all groups in the past had access to treatments promoted by medical practitioners, and some had reasons to mistrust institutional care. It follows that alternative models of healing have always been significant to communities, especially those who have been historically excluded from professional care, overwhelmingly suffer poor health outcomes, are distrustful of mainstream medicine, and wish to maintain autonomy over their bodies.

The archaeological examples that Reifschneider assembles in this book demonstrate why the inequities built into the current healthcare system are not inevitable; they are an outgrowth of the professionalization of the field of medicine, a widespread American ethos of individualism, and policies and practices that have excluded disenfranchised communities from advantageous participation in a professional healthcare system. My mother, Josephine Nassaney, recounts a time when I (Michael) suffered from a persistent high fever as a toddler in the late 1950s. To assuage my condition, my maternal grandmother, a Syrian immigrant, prepared a noxious-smelling concoction that she smeared on my chest. She had probably learned this procedure from her mother in Aleppo since nonprofessional medicine has historically been performed in the domestic sphere, predominately by women, who were trained by family or community members. When the pediatrician finally arrived for his home visit, he was met at the door with the fumes from my treatment, immediately expressed his horror at this alien home care, and informed my mother of its inferiority compared to his medicine. There was no doubt that medical practice was a power-laden field. My fever soon subsided, but whether due to the professional or folk treatment, I cannot say.

Historical archaeology demonstrates the importance of self-care as early as the eighteenth century; it is not a recent phenomenon. "Self-help" or self-care systems are often enacted outside the direct purview of state administrators and healthcare professionals and appear as James Scott's "hidden transcripts" that are accessible through materiality. Thus, archaeology is well positioned to examine the intersections between mainstream and alternative health modalities in the past and assess how alternative systems remain vital to communities that are prevented from, or choose to avoid, accessing professionalized medicine in the present.

While patients often used complementary and alternative medicine (CAM) according to Reifschneider, home care was generally rejected by formal medical practitioners who viewed it as ineffective, "primitive," and dangerous. Yet, alternative forms of care and treatment were significant for racialized, gendered, and minoritized people who did not have access to professional care, distrusted the professional medical community, and/or viewed their bodies, their health and well-being, and their care in ways that did not align with professional medicine. Historical archaeology can aid in promoting a contemporary understanding of CAM and integrative medicines by demonstrating alternative healing's long history in the United States.

Reifschneider presents a novel archaeological perspective on American healthcare and medical practice that carefully traces the long-standing relationships within the US healthcare system between medicine, health, and philosophies of freedom. Enlisting archaeological evidence—from pharmaceutical bottles, medical implements, and skeletal trauma to traces of herbal remedies, infectious lesions, and parasites recovered from privy deposits—Reifschneider connects the history of American health and medicine to discourses about individualism, citizenship, and scientific knowledge, and beliefs about hygiene, infectious disease, and patient-centered care. This book makes several original contributions to the field of historical archaeology, particularly in providing a long-term social history of the US healthcare system. Her work explicitly lays the groundwork for the nascent field of medical archaeology and also contributes case studies that intersect with emerging conversations about the archaeology of disability.

Foundational studies in medical archaeology were overwhelmingly descriptive and failed to appreciate the rich bodies of evidence that indicate "alternative" (i.e., nonscientific, and nonbiomedical) ways of achieving well-being. For example, archaeological research demonstrates how Puritan anxieties concerning bodily and spiritual decline shaped the lived experiences and material lives of the Harvard community in Cambridge, Massachusetts. Remains of pharmaceutical bottles, macrobotanical remains, clothing items, and smoking pipes suggest a rich history of healing practices employed at Harvard. Coin charms were used on the body to protect against sin and illness, while smoking tobacco was thought to be an efficient cure for cancer and respiratory illness. Indeed, archaeologists recognize that various plant species may have been used to meet the spiritual, nutritional, *and* psychosocial health needs of a community, instead of attempting to differentiate plants as *either* food *or* medicine.

Licensed physicians used what may have been seen as ineffective and physically traumatic treatments, and they were often reluctant to care for poor or marginalized people. Historical archaeological research reveals the importance of so-called alternative therapies for racialized or ethnic minorities who are more likely to undergo discrimination and other negative experiences within the conventional medical system. Archaeological evidence of medicine vials, opium-smoking paraphernalia, kegs for storing tea, and implements used to perform skin scraping and skin modification indicate Chinese railroad workers made healthcare choices that reflected a basic knowledge of Chinese medical theory and practice in conjunction with European and American patent medicines.

Archaeological material recovered from the Alabama household of a Black midwife includes animal remains, medicine bottles, foods, and tools that can be used to interpret the experiences of pregnancy and birth. African American midwives did not distinguish between spiritual and bodily health and often integrated care practices from different cultural traditions, including those rooted in African philosophies, Enlightenment theories of hygiene and medicine, and magical practices shared with Euro-American healers.

Similarly, enslaved people at Poplar Forest, Virginia, relied on ethnobotanical knowledge for nutrition and healing purposes, along with aspects of spiritual care, as evidenced by the recovery of crystals and other minerals used in conjuring practices. Community-based healthcare strategies were fundamental to various racialized and economically disadvantaged communities who could not access physician care or who were distrustful of trained and licensed doctors, as indicated by significant quantities of glass medicine bottles and healthcare equipment recovered from the Wayman African Methodist Episcopal Church in Bloomington, Illinois. Archaeologists who have examined health-seeking practices and medicinal systems among Native Americans in the wake of European colonization have observed bird bone tubes associated with healing practices and the adoption of European clothing to protect against infectious diseases.

Self-treatment was repopularized during the 1820s–1860s as "anti-authoritarian" approaches to medicine, which were fueled by anti-elitism and a general distrust of educated, middle- and upper-class professionals. Case studies in this book demonstrate how alternative medicines offered patients agency over their bodies and their care. During the nineteenth and early twentieth centuries, proprietary medicines in particular provided an important source of self-medication for individuals who were excluded or avoided professional care. Archaeological research demonstrates how a robust patent medicine market helped patients overcome negative health outcomes, deal with poverty and discrimination, and seek out alternatives to an increasingly exclusionary professional medical field.

As many of the archaeological examples in this book demonstrate, the development of the American healthcare system is historically rooted in social, political, and economic structures of inequality that exacerbate poor health outcomes in women, children, racialized minorities, immigrants, and other marginalized social groups. The closure of a number of prominent Black colleges in the late nineteenth century severely limited the role and presence of Black doctors in American medical practice. Disparities created by unequal access to professional medical care and to medical training programs encouraged members of marginalized social groups to seek care via alternative means. In addition to these structural and economic constraints, many people avoided professionally educated and trained doctors for personal reasons. These included doctors' use of radical and invasive treatments on their patients, centuries of discriminatory and racist scientific theories of medicine and the body, and citizens' pervasive distrust of medical elitism. As historical and archaeological case studies demonstrate, alternative methods of care were developed by communities that perceived a need to circumvent professional medicine.

Archaeological research also underscores the professional medical community's demand for new medical technologies and *materia medica,* or medical objects, substances, and instruments. For example, tools associated with dissection and anatomization that were foundational to the development of professional medicine during the nineteenth century have been recovered in archaeological contexts, along with human body parts that testify to early experimentation with human cadavers. Medical practice extended to various institutions seemingly unrelated to healthcare, such as the military, where the US Army managed the hygiene habits and moral characters of enlisted soldiers. The case study of the Presidio barracks of San Francisco reveals the complex interplay between citizenship, morality, and healthcare for soldiers during the late nineteenth and early twentieth centuries. Objects recovered from the barracks include patent and over-the-counter medicines, hygiene products, and recreational drugs, which inform on the relationship between Army standards of hygiene and healthcare and enlisted men's self-care practices. Analysis of artifacts from the Presidio demonstrate how enlisted soldiers often resisted or altered Army healthcare guidelines, and thus the conditions of military citizenship, by using specific products in their daily self-care routines.

In the realm of public health, the asylum was an institution developed by medical professionals during the nineteenth century to provide housing, care, and treatment for mentally ill patients. Asylums were meant to physically isolate mentally ill individuals from the broader society and relieve families of caretaking duties. Health reforms in the late nineteenth century led to transformations in patient treatment. Evidence from the Kalamazoo State Hospital Colony Farm (Michigan), for example, demonstrates how the cottage model of psychiatric care exposed patients to nature and engaged them in useful tasks and regular work routines (milking cows, harvesting fruit, tending orchards). The healing qualities of sunlight, clean air, and healthy food were effective and more humane forms of therapy.

Conversely, historical archaeological research has shown that medical science and medical research have often been cruel in their use of historically racialized, classed, and gendered bodies in unethical and violent ways. For instance, the medical establishment frequently used poor and Black bodies without consent for its own scientific advancement and the development of medical theories. These historical legacies of exploitation and discrimination are ingrained in the collective consciousness of Black and other marginalized communities. Contemporary distrust in the professional medical community among these groups inhibits care-seeking behavior and compromises medical care in the present.

Much of the archaeological research synthesized in this book focuses on how medical institutions reinforce normative standards of health and the physical body, how social conditions of inequality shape the health outcomes of marginalized communities, and how marginalized social groups develop counter-hegemonic healing practices and culturally salient medicinal systems. Reifschneider discusses many significant developments in American medical science and practice and demonstrates how historical archaeologists have contributed to our broader understanding of these key moments of transition.

Because citizenship and democratic participation were granted based on a set of relations between the individual and the state, becoming a good citizen meant maintaining standards of health and hygiene that were institutionally defined. The current US healthcare system is an outcome of the professionalization and increasing specialization of the medical field over the previous three centuries. Thus it behooves us to understand medicine and healthcare in the past if we are to chart a path for future well-being for all who aim to participate in the American experience.

Michael S. Nassaney, *Founding Series Editor*

Krysta Ryzewski, *Series Coeditor*

ACKNOWLEDGMENTS

I would like to acknowledge numerous people for their important roles in writing this book, although there are too many to name here. I would first like to extend my sincere gratitude to Michael Nassaney for encouraging me to undertake this project for the series and for his guidance in developing the manuscript. I would similarly like to thank Krysta Ryzewski for her continued support and assistance throughout the writing process. I am especially grateful to Mary Puckett for her continued patience and hard work in helping this book come to fruition. I would also like to thank Kristen Fellows, Stephen Brighton, and an anonymous reviewer for their constructive comments on previous drafts of the manuscript. A huge thank-you to Annalisa Bolin, for her keen intellect and editorial expertise.

I would like to recognize Suzy Fish, Paul Fish, and Charles Adams, who introduced me to the wonders of archaeology over 20 years ago. I thank them for believing in me and supporting my burgeoning academic journey. I am infinitely thankful to my mentor, Barb Voss, whose incredible research continues to inspire me. She has taught me the importance of theoretical and empirical rigor and has provided generous guidance throughout my career. Special thanks are due to the Presidio Trust, particularly Liz Melicker and Kari Jones, for supporting my research on the Presidio Building 104 materials.

This acknowledgment would not be complete without recognizing the incredible dedication of my students at San Francisco State University. In particular, I would like to thank my exceptional students, RJ Stevens and Clay Kirkwood, for their hard work and expertise on the Presidio project. I thank my colleagues in the Department of Anthropology at SFSU, as well as faculty members of the STS Hub, who provided assistance and guidance throughout the writing process. Many thanks to Martha Lincoln for her inspiring conversations and for holding me accountable to our regular writing "Zoom dates" during the pandemic. A heartfelt thanks to friends, family, and my spouse, Stephen Levendusky, for their continued love and support.

1

Introduction

I am writing this book amid the ongoing COVID-19 pandemic, arguably the most widespread and significant epidemic event to affect global populations during the last century. On December 30, 2019, a bronchial sample from a patient tested positive with pan-betacoronavirus (COVID-19) (Fauci et al. 2020). Like other coronaviruses, such as severe acute respiratory syndrome (SARS), COVID-19 is a highly contagious virus (Yuki et al. 2020). The spread of COVID-19 across the world since late 2019 has spurred a series of emergency measures on the part of national and international political committees and public health organizations (Stratton 2020). The COVID-19 pandemic has had a lasting, deep impact on human health and has permeated every facet of social, economic, and political life for billions of people. In the United States, the pandemic exacerbated the preexisting high costs of healthcare, inequitable insurance coverage, and poor health outcomes, further demonstrating that the US healthcare system has failed to provide cohesive coverage to American populations compared to other developed countries (Blank 2012; Blank et al. 2018). In addition, American healthcare policies have historically failed to address disparities in social health determinants such as education, living conditions, employment, and access to quality care (Ahmed et al. 2001; Marmot 2005; Syme 2004).

Responses to the pandemic clearly revealed these deep fault lines in American medicine, reflecting institutional incompetence, discriminatory policies, and a lack of centralized healthcare management, all of which redoubled the effects of health disparities that already existed. Those without medical insurance or reliable access to clinical care were disproportionately affected by COVID-19, suffering from higher morbidity and mortality rates (Bambra et al. 2020; Mishra et al. 2021; van Dorn et al. 2020). Overfilled hospitals, inadequate medical staffing, and limited access to vaccines and drugs were a few indicators of the fallibility of the US healthcare system (Rydland et al. 2022). Furthermore, the lack of centralized, cohesive, and federally initiated public health policies to control the spread of the virus, especially in the early stages of the pandemic, suggest that the scoping of prospective impacts and potential solutions was politically inadequate (Bergquist et al. 2020). Instead, public health responses to COVID-19 were often under the aegis of state and local governments due to a lack of national reporting, planning, and policy implementation (Xu and Basu 2020). Moreover, the pandemic showed how certain bodies came to matter. Ad hoc triage measures that sought to protect the lives of some while facilitating the deaths of others aggravated preexisting socioeconomic inequalities—what Mbembe (2008) has famously termed "necropolitics." Vulnerable communities most affected by the lack of state protections include communities of color, elderly individuals, those with preexisting or chronic health conditions, and low-income employees who were disproportionately exposed to the disease (ironically termed "essential workers") (Bowleg 2020).

COVID-19 responses also brought into stark reality the overt politicization of clinical medicine and public health arenas. COVID-19 responses exposed, if not deepened, public distrust of doctors and professional medicine. Elected leaders, most (in)famously Donald Trump, took advantage of public anti-elitism by promoting a language of "medical populism" and partisanship (Lasco 2020). These leaders minimized the severity of the pandemic, spread medical misinformation, and endorsed conspiracy theories; they encouraged a general distrust of federal and state officials along with government agencies and promoted a fear of the "deep state" (Eberl et al. 2021). Poignant examples include criticisms of the practice of face masking as well as anti-vaccination campaigns, which were disastrously reframed in terms of individual liberty and anti-government intervention (Earnshaw et al. 2020). But this contemporary distrust of medical authority and the sociopolitical backlash against public health institutions (such as the World Health Organization [WHO] and Centers for Disease Control and Prevention [CDC]) within the context of the COVID-19 pandemic are not recent occurrences. Instead, they are strikingly similar to Jacksonian era anti-elitism and the "do it yourself" ethos of household medicine during the nineteenth century.

Responses to COVID-19 were foundationally shaped by the American experience of healthcare and medicine through time. Examining wellness and medicine through the lens of archaeology, this book aims to illuminate genealogies of medical practice and politics and the ways Americans' experiences reflect and negotiate with these historical dynamics. While a full review of the COVID-19 pandemic and its innumerable responses and effects is outside the scope of this book, it is impossible to synthesize archaeological literature on healthcare and medicine without viewing it through the lens of this pandemic. It is equally impossible to theorize current pandemic responses without a deep understanding of American medical history and the material instantiations of public health and medicine. The recent pandemic poses timely—and timeless—questions that are suitable for archaeological inquiry: What are the tenuous and complex relationships between the scientific and medical community, politicians and government agencies, and citizens? Whose lives are deemed valuable and in need of protection, and whose are considered expendable? How are these decisions made? How is access to healthcare overdetermined by social and political factors? How are these patterns of access to care exacerbated in times of health crisis? How are seemingly nonpolitical medical interventions and public health measures politicized, and with what effects? How are these varying practices and ideologies materialized, and how do they play out on individual bodies? How can archaeology show the contemporary healthcare system's historical roots in specific regulatory and political forces that continue to have significant material and bodily effects?

The discipline of historical archaeology is well suited to address questions regarding the American experience of medicine and healthcare. Like the field of archaeology more generally, historical archaeology examines the human condition via the analysis of artifacts, or material culture. In North American intellectual spheres, historical archaeology has developed its own unique research methods and research orientations and agendas over the past seventy or so years. Historical archaeology has variously been defined by a specific temporal emphasis, as embodying a unique set of research methods, and as having a distinctive research focus. When defined by its temporal focus, historical archaeology includes the study of the post-contact world, which in North America correlates generally to the fifteenth century onward (Deetz 2010). Researchers considered Europeans, or colonial populations, as *historic,* while Native, colonized populations were termed *prehistoric.* These boundaries between *prehistoric* and *historic* have more recently been criticized for relegating Native people to a timeless, primitive past (Lightfoot 1995; Silliman 2005). Today, historical archaeologists take a broad temporal approach by examining historical processes and their material outcomes.

In terms of methodology, historical archaeologists combine independent lines of evidence (Wylie 2000). These include oral histories, ethnohistories, visual representations, artifacts, and myriad textual documents, which in combination help to develop robust, empirically grounded narratives of the past. As a thematic orientation, historical archaeologists investigate the social and political processes that define the modern world: large-scale urbanization, mercantilism and capitalism, globalization, and contact between different cultures (Hall and Silliman 2009, Orser 2010). While historical archaeology tends to defy any coherent, agreed upon, and singular definition, Orser (2016: 16) defines it as "a multi-disciplinary field that shares a special relationship with the formal disciplines of anthropology and history, focuses its attention on the post-Columbian past, and seeks to understand the global nature of modern life."

With roots in historic preservation, early historical archaeological studies in the United States tended to focus on European contexts and sites of "national significance" such as Thomas Jefferson's Monticello and George Washington's Mount Vernon. By the 1970s, studies underwent a distinct paradigm shift. Historical archaeologists used their access to vast sources of written and unwritten information to reconstruct the histories of individuals and communities who had been largely left out of the official narratives of American history: women, children, laborers, immigrants, people of color, Native Americans, and others who did not fit neatly into the normative, mainstream standards of the time. Today, historical archaeology has a strong social justice bent; by telling the stories of marginalized people throughout history, we can address past injustices and chart more equitable futures in the present.

Historical archaeology has a long and robust history of investigating healthcare practices, medical institutions, medicalization, public health, and medical philosophies. Recent scholarship has adopted critical, socially engaged approaches to examining medicine and healthcare. Various thematic frames have proven useful here: topics include but are not limited to archaeological studies of ethnomedical traditions (Linn 2010; Wilkie 1996a), community-based healthcare (Cabak et al. 1995), reproductive health (Barnes 2021), medical institutions (Scott 2023), medical consumerism and medicalization (Barnes 2023; Lee 2017; Verstraete 2023), and the sociopolitics of healthcare and public health (Camp et al. 2023; Larsen 1994; Smith 2007). Historical archaeologists have addressed these key themes, and others, through the lenses of gender, sexuality, class, race, and more recently, disability. The goal of this book is not to survey the history of the American medical profession per se (see Starr 2017 for a comprehensive review), but to touch upon significant developments in American medical science and practice and demonstrate how historical archaeologists have contributed to our broader understanding of these key moments of transition. Given the diversity, complexity, and volume of these different veins of scholarship on American healthcare, I divided the chapters in this book into themes that highlight historical archaeologists' critical methodological and topical contributions.

These chapters include: the history of medical science and healthcare professionalization, including the coterminous growth of alternative medicine; healthcare consumerism; and public health and sanitary reform. Each chapter synthesizes important historical debates while simultaneously showing how historical archaeological research contributes to and complicates these conversations. This scholarship has significantly advanced our understanding of how medical science and healthcare policies are implemented or modified *on the ground* by tacking between macro- and microscales of analysis. Historical archaeologists have proven adept at examining "local" phenomena couched within "extra-local" and "global" contexts, heeding Orser's (1996) calls for multiscalar methodologies within the discipline. The archaeological scholarship examined in this book demonstrates the usefulness of multiscalar approaches by showing what people *do* to maintain their health and care for others, while simultaneously exploring the broader social politics that inform local healthcare ideologies and localized medical practices. Throughout this book, I show how house deposits, middens, latrines, hospital waste pits, and other archaeological deposits may be interpreted as micro-scale sites of healthcare policy implementation; these refuse deposits provide a cumulative record of practices, which in turn are structured by—and structure in turn—broader social processes (compare with Bourdieu 1977). Finally, thematic discussions in this book highlight how historical archaeologists have used material culture, archives, and ethnography to highlight how many structural health inequalities in the past continue to marginalize certain social groups in the present. As many of the archaeological examples in this book demonstrate, the development of the American healthcare system is historically rooted in social, political, and economic structures of inequality that exacerbate poor health outcomes in women, children, racialized minorities, immigrants, and other marginalized social groups (Dickman et al. 2017).

Studying the dynamics of power in healthcare practices requires that scholars explore how state- and institution-sponsored policies affect the body, health, and health-seeking behaviors at individual and community levels. The practice of medicine and the implementation of healthcare policies are never apolitical acts. Rather, broader political and social systems always inform medicine and healthcare. Given the dialogical nature between healthcare and society, this book foregrounds archaeological scholarship that interrogates the complex relationships between medicine, authority, power, and resistance. Historical archaeological research has contributed to broader knowledge concerning the role of healthcare institutions in shaping new practices and subjectivities (Smith 2007). Other studies demonstrate the degree to which collective modes of action have subverted or altered dominant healthcare systems. Much of the archaeological research synthesized in this book focuses on how medical institutions reinforce normative standards of health and the physical body, how social conditions of inequality shape the health outcomes of marginalized communities, and how marginalized social groups develop counter-hegemonic healing practices and culturally salient medicinal systems.

Throughout the book, I demonstrate how broad healthcare mandates and directives affect the intimate spheres of healthcare practice. Each chapter begins with a discussion of macro-scale events, such as institutional reforms, and goes on to examine archaeological case studies that demonstrate how these macro-scale events in American medicine shape individuals' healthcare experiences on the ground.

Chapter 2 traces the history of professional medical spheres and explores the boundaries between professional and nonprofessional medical sectors, showing how both fields of medicine constituted loosely defined realms of practice that were guided by broader sociopolitical arrangements, including economic access and social identification. Health interventions were shaped by competing metaphorical, scientific, and sociohistorical understandings of disease (Lupton 1993). These tensions played out at both local and national levels, involving health organizations, physicians, Progressive Era reformers, and the communities that were targeted by health policies. Archaeological research shows how racialized, immigrant, and other marginalized communities resisted top-down public health measures and developed alternative modes of preventative and community health that accommodated community health needs. "Self-help" or self-care systems were often enacted outside the direct purview of state administrators and healthcare professionals, thus constituting what Scott (2008) refers to as "hidden transcripts." The focus on materiality gives us access to these hidden transcripts. This archaeological work is significant in that by examining the intersections between mainstream and alternative health modalities in the past, we are better positioned to address how alternative systems remain vital to communities that are prevented from, or choose to avoid, accessing professionalized medicine in the present. By addressing diverse health-seeking behaviors in the past and showing how different communities have engaged with the professional medical sphere over time, historical archaeologists have made important contributions that meaningfully reflect onto our current healthcare landscape.

Archaeological examinations of consumer trends in medicine similarly highlight the relationship between self-care and institutionalized medicine, but within the context of the market. In Chapter 3, I show how the emergence of new medical marketplaces allowed patients to identify as medical consumers, while patients' growing distrust of professional medicine shaped emergent consumer trends during the nineteenth century. A burgeoning proprietary medicine market and new forms of medical advertising reached a literate audience that was receptive to the integration of medicine with market forces (Young 2015). Drug advertising simultaneously medicalized certain bodily conditions and generated a perceived need for drugs to cure these newfound afflictions (Conrad and Leiter 2008). Archaeological studies reveal that people's engagement with medicine *shapes* and *is shaped by* their social and political worlds (Barnes 2015; Linn 2010; Wilkie 1996a, 1996b). This archaeological research also shows how medicalization—the process by which normal bodily conditions become pathologized through drug development and advertising—affected how people understood their physical realities. By addressing patterns of medicine consumption and consumerism, historical archaeologists have shown the pharmaceutical industry's role in establishing health ideals and influencing subjective understandings of health, illness, and the body. As archaeologists have cogently noted, medical consumerism and direct-to-consumer advertising (DTCA) are not new contemporary phenomena but rather an outgrowth of advertising and consumer trends of the nineteenth century (Barnes 2023). Furthermore, as these shifts continued, the wide availability of proprietary drugs and drug advertisements enabled patient autonomy from the professional medical field and resulted in diverse household and community-based healthcare systems (Segal 2020).

Chapter 4 reviews archaeologies of public health. Many of the studies in this chapter show how regulatory agencies deemed some populations more at risk and more contagious—riskier—than others (Bashford 2002; Brown 2009). Those populations that were considered contagious by virtue of their citizenship status, race, ethnicity, sexuality, or gender were often forcibly institutionalized, unequally targeted by public health reforms, or excluded from participation in civil society. Studies of the relationship between social life and civic belonging, spurred by Foucault's impactful work, or the relationship between life and politics (Foucault 1990, 2010), have been central to academic inquiry. While Foucault's work on biopolitics has not been integrated into archaeology on the far-reaching scale seen in other disciplines (but see Cowie 2011), much historical archaeological work problematizes the encounter between life and politics, particularly within the context of public healthcare and administration. Historical archaeologists have historicized contemporary understandings of public health, sanitation, and hygiene. In doing so, they have explored the deep political structures of these medical contexts and shown how life-sustaining practices operate through a nexus of biopower, particularly the regulation of individual subjects by the state. Regulatory structures frequently operate through institutions, agencies, and other organizations that mobilize virtue discourses and promote individualized and normative understandings of health and the body (Camp et al. 2023). In turn, these discourses construct subjects who have a vested material interest in maintaining the terms of political belonging. Contexts of enslavement and other forms of institutionalization (including hospitals, sanatoria, and asylums) have proven fruitful for archaeological explorations of public health interventions and different—even competing—metaphorical, scientific, and sociohistorical understandings of disease.

Biopolitical discourses and their attendant material practices help differentiate between those who are and are not acceptable sorts of individual beings within a broader moral/medical schema (Halse 2012). This process of individualizing the collective mass has the effect of increasing management at the individual human level, but it also effectively erases one's personal identity in order to "inscribe a new persona—that of the (virtuous) bio-citizen" (Halse 2012: 50). *Biocitizenship* proves a useful concept for examining the relationships between health status, citizenship status, and rights. Chapter 4 concludes by examining archaeological and historical research on the intersection between tuberculosis, institutionalization, and citizenship in nineteenth-century northern California. As the studies at the end of this chapter demonstrate, citizenship and democratic participation were granted based on a set of relations between the individual and the state: in these, the individual actively strove to improve the overall well-being of the state (Halse 2012: 50), and their conduct reflected certain "regimes of truth" (Rose 1999: 19). Becoming a good (virtuous) biological citizen meant maintaining standards of health that were institutionally defined. While Rose (1999) positions this political rationality in the mid-twentieth century, historical archaeologists have demonstrated the intimate relationship between "good" citizenship and health during the nineteenth century as well as the twentieth.

The archaeological scholarship discussed in Chapter 5 examines the intersections between seemingly disparate, yet interconnected, elements of medical theory and practice. Specifically, I highlight the tensions between regulatory medicine and self-care by focusing on my research into enlisted soldiers' healthcare practices at the Presidio of San Francisco. This case study foregrounds the complex interplay between citizenship, morality, and healthcare for soldiers at the Presidio during the late nineteenth and early twentieth centuries. The study uses "biocitizenship" as a guiding concept to explore how the US Army managed the healthcare behaviors of enlisted soldiers in this period, focusing on their hygiene habits and moral characters.

The idea of biocitizenship explains the process through which citizenship status becomes linked to states of biological existence (Rose and Novas 2005). During the late nineteenth century, US Army War Department and Health Department policies were influenced by Progressive Era discourses concerning biological identification and standardized ideals of hygiene, sexuality, and morality (Bristow 1996; Shah 2001). During the late nineteenth and early twentieth centuries, citizenship status was conferred not only through race, economic status, and birth rights, but also via the health statuses that these social identities came to represent (Ong et al. 1996). As Wald (2020: 193) notes, the health of the nation marked the power of the nation and the body politic; health concerns could be recast as a call to public action and a reaffirmation of national potential. At the turn of the twentieth century, the US Army War Department and Health Department developed hygiene and healthcare programs to shape a "new type of soldier" and thus a new type of American citizen (Bristow 1996). This study focuses on artifacts that were used in personal care practices, including patent and over-the-counter (OTC) medicines, hygiene products, and recreational drugs. I use these items to examine the relationship between Army standards of hygiene and healthcare and enlisted men's self-care practices. The results of the study demonstrate that enlisted soldiers at the Presidio often resisted or altered Army healthcare guidelines, and thus the conditions of military citizenship, by using specific products in their daily self-care routines.

As the archaeological examples in this book demonstrate, the inequities that are built into the current healthcare system are not inevitable; they are an outgrowth of the professionalization of the field of medicine, a widespread American ethos of individualism, and policies and practices that have excluded marginalized and minoritized communities from advantageous participation in a professional healthcare system (Baker et al. 2008; Matthew 2018; Singh et al. 2017). Historical archaeological research shows that medical science and medical research have historically used racialized, classed, and gendered bodies in unethical and violent ways (Cooper Owens 2017; Savitt 1982; Washington 2006). Across the eighteenth through twentieth centuries, physicians and medical institutions participated in a long-standing tradition of discriminating against women, immigrants, impoverished populations, and Black Americans. The medical establishment frequently used poor and Black bodies without consent for its own scientific advancement and the development of medical theories (Halperin 2007; Nystrom 2014). These historical legacies of exploitation and discrimination are ingrained in the collective consciousness of Black and other marginalized communities. Contemporary distrust in the professional medical community among these groups inhibits care-seeking behavior and compromises medical care in the present (Corbie-Smith et al. 2002). A holistic understanding of the mechanisms of power in healthcare and medicine requires that scholars attend not only to dominant structures, but also to patients' resistance to power and authority.

Studying the US healthcare system over the past 300 years contextualizes America's current diverse therapeutic landscape. Chapters in this book detail the professionalization of the medical field and simultaneously account for therapeutic practices that lie outside mainstream medicine. Alternative medicines, herbalism, and other homeopathic techniques did not arise "phoenixlike" in America over the past few decades (Johnston 2004). Neither did homeopathic therapies, spiritual healing, and Afrocentric healing practices, to name a few, disappear during the establishment of scientific, mainstream medicine. Instead, alternative models of healing have always been significant to communities that have been historically excluded from professional care, that overwhelmingly suffer poor health outcomes, or that are distrustful of mainstream medicine and wish to maintain autonomy over their bodies (Eisenberg et al. 1998; Johnston 2004). Archaeological research shows how alternative medicines in the form of herbal or proprietary drugs were important curative and therapeutic resources for most American households regardless of race, class, or gender. Even seemingly nonmedicinal goods, such as soda water, had psychological and bodily therapeutic effects for marginalized communities (Linn 2010).

The conclusion of this book foregrounds the contemporary significance of archaeological research on medical professionalization and alternative therapies. Contemporary clinical discourses tend to disregard the meaningfulness of alternative therapeutic practices for patient well-being. Often, these discourses relegate alternative medicines to a subaltern status and/or frame patients' use of alternative medicines as a form of "noncompliance" (Ning 2013). CAM was theorized by clinicians and social scientists in the 1970s–1990s as patient "resistance"; more recent work in anthropology and clinical medicine has conceptualized alternative medicine practitioners as medical "designers" or "bricoleurs" capable of creating plural healthcare traditions (Bates 2000; Bivins 2013; Johnston 2004). Rather than explore the effectiveness of alternative medicine per se, I argue that historical archaeology can aid in promoting a contemporary understanding of CAM and integrative medicines by demonstrating alternative healing's long history in the United States. Careful attention to historical and archaeological contexts also shows the foundations of alternative medicines in community distrust of, or exclusion from, mainstream clinical medicine. This work highlights the broader inequities of the professional field of medicine while also showcasing the agency of communities that develop healthcare systems that work for their members. Examples include research on Irish American community care (Linn 2010) and African American care networks in homes and churches (Cabak et al. 1995). Many of the archaeological studies highlighted in this book complicate the very idea of "alternative medicine" as something truly marginal (Ning 2013). For many individuals and social groups, healing traditions rooted in localized and lay knowledge systems proliferated both *in spite of* and *because of* the professionalization of medicine from the eighteenth to twentieth centuries.

Finally, this book calls for archaeologists to critically assess how certain disciplinary concepts guide archaeological research on healthcare and how these define the kinds of questions that we ask about the past. Throughout this book, I argue that medicine frequently operates as a disciplinary force and as a means of "power over life" (Foucault et al. 1997). Public health institutions and medical establishments mobilize two poles of biopower: first, through the individual, creating subjects who understand themselves as medicalized selves (Lupton 1997), and second, on a population level, through technologies of normalization and control. Foucault's work on biopower has provided an invaluable tool for interrogating the techniques by which bodies have been controlled and commodified through medical practices. But recently, anthropologists have critically addressed the insufficiency of biopolitical frameworks for contending with the varied goals, substance, and social nature of the medical encounter (Buch 2014, 2015; Smith-Morris 2018; Yates-Doerr 2012). As Yates-Doerr states of her own research on weight loss programs, "Power is important, but a different framework is also needed: one that considers medical practices that operate amid constraints of hierarchy and control, employing compassion, concern, and relationality" (2012: 137). Institutions and regulatory agencies often impose health paradigms on subjects, yet exchanges in clinical settings often disregard institutional protocols and instead direct attention toward specific context-dependent desires and needs of patients and providers. I argue that we need archaeological paradigms that explore the *excesses* of care: ones that attend to moments in care that exceed biopolitical paradigms of power and authority. Care often involves directed preventative measures and treatments, but also entails forms of acknowledgment that support individual and community well-being. Archaeological investigations that stress the importance of affect and emotion may bring us closer to understanding the personal, *careful,* and *caring* relationships that develop in the medical encounter.

2

Professional Medicine and Archaeologies of the American Healthcare System

The current US healthcare system is an outcome of the professionalization and increasing specialization of the medical field over the previous three centuries (Ayo 2012; Starr 2009). University-educated physicians, the development of medical institutions like the American Medical Association (AMA), state and federal legislative reforms, and healthcare insurance regulations have shaped American medicine since the late eighteenth century (Starr 2017). The professionalization of medicine is a recent development in the United States compared to European countries like Germany, Denmark, and France, which had developed centrally administered healthcare systems by the early eighteenth century (Berg 2010; Ramsey 2002; Vallgårda 1995). Equally significant are the ways that patients responded to the nascent professional medical field in the United States. This chapter focuses on the histories of two parallel veins of medical practice, one that may be called "allopathic" or scientific medicine and other alternative or heterodox healthcare systems.[1] Despite attempts over the past two centu-

---

1 Throughout this book, I use the term *alternative* to refer to medical practices that do not include scientific medicine, biomedicine, or medical epistemologies and ontologies that are taught in university settings. When discussing contemporary alternative medical systems, I use *CAM (complementary and alternative medicine),* which is the term most often used in academic and clinical settings. Other terms used by social scientists and clinicians for scientific medicine include *allopathic medicine, biomedicine, mainstream medicine, Western medicine,* and *regular medicine.* Alternative medicine includes herbalism, hydropathy, chiropractic, osteopathy, aromatherapy, cultural healing systems such as Chinese traditional medicine, and any other organized medicinal system that does not include scientific training or practice. Other terms commonly used to describe alternative medicine include folk medicine, domestic medicine, quackery, irregular medicine, and Indigenous medicine. I further note that the terms used by healthcare providers and patients to designate *mainstream* biomedicine and CAM as opposing dualities are problematic. These naming exercises reflect the perceived dominance of *Western* biomedicine internationally and may also be the result of historical constructivism, rather

ries by legal organizations, medical institutions, and practicing physicians to create a cohesive, streamlined, and professional network of medicine, American healthcare has always constituted a diverse therapeutic landscape. Archaeological research demonstrates the utility of examining medical objects and everyday practices; its studies show how professional medical institutions, ideologies, and mandates affected people's most intimate lives.

Archaeologists have traced scientific medicine, or biomedicine, as only one of many coexisting models of care. The existence of pluralistic healthcare practices within America speaks to the different ways in which people thought about their bodies, and the numerous roles that pharmaceuticals, material objects, plants, and animals played in treatment (Bonasera and Raymer 2001; Sutherland et al. 2013; Voeks 1993; Wilkie 1996b, 2003). Archaeologists have also examined models of health around a range of axes, from biophysical fitness to community belonging to spiritual wellness (Bonasera and Raymer 2001; Sutherland et al. 2013; Voeks 1993; Wilkie 1996b, 2003). For example, many healers in the African diaspora interpreted health within the context of bodily, spiritual, and mental well-being; thus, healing practices targeted the whole being, not just the corporeal body (Wilkie 2000). Herbal remedies used by various Native American communities similarly cured symptoms and elevated one's bodily and spiritual self (Hutchinson 2022). Native Americans and African Americans exchanged botanical knowledge, thus creating a diverse repertoire of ethnobotanical practices (Wilkie 1996a).

Medicine constitutes a loosely defined "boundary object" (Star and Griesemer 1989) of practice that is characterized by broader sociopolitical structures, including economic access and social identification. "Medicine" itself is a fuzzy category that acts as a mediator between different social worlds. In this sense, the perceived epistemological boundaries between scientific/mainstream and alternative medicine change depending on social and political circumstances. Finally, medicine performs the work of connecting diverse individuals together, including experts (doctors) and laypersons (patients). This results in a multidimensional milieu of interconnected material practices.

---

than representative of a manifest reality. Moreover, *alternative and complementary* implies a sense of moral authority: it is *alternative* to something, in most cases the absence of biomedicine/scientific medicine (Gale 2014). Despite these linguistic issues, I attempt to use emic terms that practitioners used/use in describing their therapeutic systems, or generally use the terms *scientific* and *alternative*.

Historical archaeology has long focused on telling the histories of marginalized people (Orser 2010). As such, historical archaeologists have played an integral role in investigating how American medical theories (Carley 1981; Fisher et al. 2007; Howson 1993) and the seemingly biological (and moral) inferiority of certain social groups (Werner and Novak 2010) have historically served to justify unequal access to professional medical care. Even after American physicians and surgeons were required to receive standard medical training to practice, patient participation in clinical and hospital care remained a privileged position. A close examination of the materiality of healthcare-related practices is important to understanding contemporary sociopolitics: by examining a range of nondominant therapies and ideologies in the past, we are better positioned to comprehend the historical roots and continuities of alternative healing in the present. By addressing the sociopolitics of health-seeking behaviors in the past and showing how diverse communities engaged with professional medicine, archaeologists have made important contributions that meaningfully reflect on our present-day realities. Historical archaeological research demonstrates that the inequities built into the current healthcare system are not inevitable but are historically rooted in these key developmental moments.

This chapter synthesizes archaeological research that reflects on the professionalization of the field of medicine from the American colonial period until the present. The goal is not to provide a comprehensive review of the history of professional medicine (see Starr 2017), but overview key developments in American medical practice and demonstrate how historical archaeologists have contributed to our broader understanding of these historical moments. The discussions are organized thematically and chronologically. The first section describes key historical moments in the professionalization of the medical field, including etiologies of disease, diagnosis, and medical treatment during each of these moments. This section also discusses medical training and licensing within the professional sector of American medicine. The second section of this chapter uses historical archaeological research to demonstrate how marginalized ethnic minorities and women negotiated the terms and conditions of the burgeoning professional medical sector. As the historical and archaeological examples in this section illustrate, alternative forms of care and treatment were significant for racialized, gendered, and minoritized people who did not have access to professional care, distrusted the professional medical community, and/or viewed their bodies, their health and well-being, and their care in ways that did not align with professional medicine. The conclusion of this chapter argues that situating the field of medicine in its social, political, and material contexts provides an important backdrop for understanding other themes within American medicine, including public health, health consumerism, and medicine in institutional settings.

The Professionalization of American Medicine: 1700s–1900s

What sociologist and medical historian Paul Starr calls "the professionalization of American medicine" (2017) took place over the course of the eighteenth, nineteenth, and twentieth centuries. Modern medicine, according to Starr (2017: 3), "is an elaborate system of specialized knowledge, technical procedures, and rules of behavior." Starr also argues that the contemporary medical field is a power-laden field of practice; it has been formed by regimes of power and authority, new medical markets, and conditions of belief and experience (Starr 2017: 4). This section presents, chronologically, key systems of knowledge, technical expertise and training, institutional developments, and power dynamics that shaped the professional sector of medical practice from the late 1700s until the early twentieth century.

Specialized Knowledge: Theories of the Body and Medical Technologies

The premises of late eighteenth- through mid-nineteenth-century medical disease and treatment among physicians were based on Hippocratic medical theory. Theories of the Hippocratic school were developed in the second century AD by Galen, the physician to Roman emperor Marcus Aurelius (Jouanna and van der Eijk 2012). Hippocratic medicine regarded disease not as a specific or localized event, but as a general imbalance in the body. The human body was formed by four humors: black bile, yellow bile, blood, and phlegm. Each of the four humoral elements—earth, water, air, and fire—manifested a different quality: dryness, coldness, heat, and moistness (Haller 1981: 4). Normal health was constituted by the balance of the four humors in the body, and any imbalance resulted in disease. Humors could be expelled or equalized through drastic physical interventions, such as venesection (bleeding) and blistering the skin, or through vomiting, urination, or defecation. "Heroic medicine," which formed the basis of medical practice during the eighteenth and nineteenth centuries in Euro-American contexts, used a range of implements and substances to facilitate the expulsion of bodily fluids in order, theoretically, to promote healing (Figure 2.1). The scalpel, or the "physician's pocket companion"

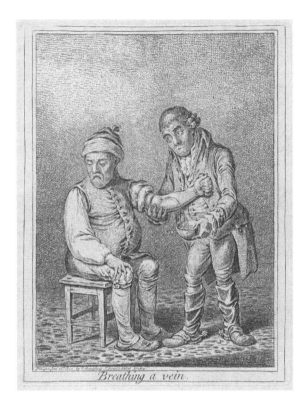

Figure 2.1. James Gillray, *Breathing a Vein*. Wikimedia Commons, CC0 1.0.

(Haller 1981: 42), was used in phlebotomy operations; blood was expelled through cuts in the wrist, head, ankle, or breast. Antimony, calomel (mercurous chloride), jalap, and rhubarb were also popular medicines used to induce vomiting, sweating, and bleeding. Although biomedical theories have replaced humoral theory in contemporary medicine, vestiges of these older ideas still exist in contemporary language. Current vernacular phrases like "feed a cold and starve a fever" and "a shock to the system" draw their meaning from humoral models of healthcare (Helman 1978).

Hippocratic theories of the body, disease, and medical treatment were generally accepted within professional medicine until the mid-nineteenth century. The seventeenth-century Scientific Revolution had little effect on medical theory and practice in Europe and Anglo-American contexts, as it did in other scientific fields such as biology, chemistry, and geology (Jewson 1974). Common limitations of knowledge and practice constrained secular medical practitioners and physicians since there was no safe way for doctors to examine the internal mechanics of the live, functioning body. Physicians either diagnosed diseases by analyzing the bodily fluids of their patients, such as blood, saliva, or urine, or relied on patients' descriptions of their symptoms (Antic and DeMay 2014). Most physicians did not have access to human bodies to examine their internal workings, nor did they study the long-term development of disease as a response to internal and external factors. Practical knowledge of the body, or what might be called "internal medicine" today, did not exist, since dissection and anatomization were illegal in most states in the United States until the 1860s. In addition, physicians rarely examined the bodies of patients during clinical encounters, but instead relied on patients' detailed descriptions of their symptoms. In short, disease was "couched in terms of the patient's complaint" (Jewson 1974: 371), not the underlying physical causes that may have influenced physiological abnormalities. Until the early nineteenth century, physicians' diagnoses foregrounded the development of complex taxonomies of disease, or *nosologies*. Diagnosis became "a chaotic compendium of syndromes extrapolated from the patient's subjective experience of 'feeling poorly'" (Jewson 1974).

The American Civil War precipitated drastic developments in medical science, particularly diagnostics and hygiene. Nearly 750,000 soldiers died during the Civil War because of infectious diseases and traumatic injuries (Devine 2016: 153). Despite high morbidity and mortality rates among soldiers, Civil War battlefields provided surgeons and physicians with clinical experiences they would not have otherwise had (Devine 2014, 2016; Key 1968). The challenges of medicine in conflict zones demanded that physicians quickly develop new scientific methods for assessing and treating soldiers. Civil War physicians were also keen to test infectious disease theories to reduce rates of fever and dysentery in the camps. Civil War surgeons were some of the first to use Joseph Lister's methods of disinfecting wounds and surgical implements (Devine 2014: 155; Trombold 2011). Army physicians and surgeons were at the forefront of emerging etiologies of disease, and often worked alongside a prestigious international medical community that included Joseph Lister, Louis Pasteur, and Robert Koch (Devine 2014). The Army Medical Department's government-sponsored research on cholera was influenced by Louis Pasteur's experiments on fermentation, and Joseph Woodward, curator of the Army Medical Museum, was in communication with Rudolf Virchow, a colleague of Robert Koch, to develop micropathological research tools and collections (Devine 2014: 154). The need for medical research to serve the military community, along

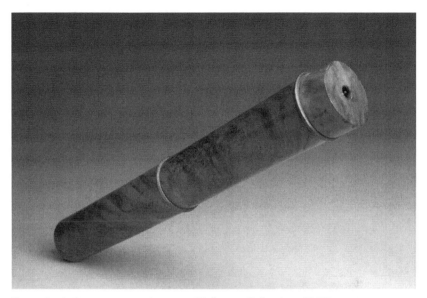

Figure 2.2. Laënnec-type stethoscope. Wellcome Collection, CC-BY-4.0.

with the necessary funding, put military medicine at the forefront of US medical science in the mid-nineteenth century.

New technological inventions also shaped medical science. The invention of the stethoscope by René Laënnec in 1816 enabled physicians to listen to the "inner workings" of a patient's lungs and hearts (Figure 2.2), and by 1818, it was applied to obstetrics to listen to fetal heart sounds (Bishop 1980: 452; Duffin 2014). Laënnec developed the original stethoscope in order to listen to one of his female patients' hearts, as rules of propriety prohibited direct application of the doctor's ear to a woman's chest (Bishop 1980).

The X-ray machine also had a profound impact on diagnosis, especially when identifying fractures and confirming the presence of foreign objects inside patients' bodies. Physicist Wilhelm Conrad Röntgen first confirmed the applicability of X-rays on a living person when he used them to take a picture of his wife's hand in 1895 (Howell 2016: 342). By 1900, physicians' use of X-ray machines, specifically in hospitals, was considered an essential tool in diagnostics and clinical care (Howell 2016). The development of percussion technologies in medicine, which date to the mid-eighteenth century in Europe and America, meant physicians could use their fingers or an instrument to tap on the surface of the body to test for abnormalities.

Physicians commonly used chest percussion techniques to listen for the presence of abdominal fluid, and doctors developed a variety of tools, such as reflex hammers, to "sound" the bodies of their patients (Lanska 1989).

Archaeological research has foregrounded the significance of the professional medical community's demand for new medical technologies and *materia medica,* or medical objects, substances, and instruments. Archaeological research carried out in New Brunswick, New Jersey, at the former residences of two doctors, Clifford Morrogh and Frank Donahue (Veit 1996), examines how new medical technologies were implemented at the local level. Both were innovative physicians and scientists during the late nineteenth and early twentieth centuries. Dr. Morrogh was one of the first physicians in the United States to use anesthesia during surgeries and, according to historical documents, his surgical successes included tying carotid arteries, removing gallstones, and treating strangulated hernias (Veit 1996: 37). Archaeological excavations at the residences of Dr. Morrogh and Dr. Donahue, a similarly innovative practitioner, uncovered medical tools and implements used in surgery, including gynecological tools, hypodermic syringes, and general practice tools. New medical technologies, like those used by Morrogh and Donahue in New Brunswick, contributed to medical science at a community level and hastened new developments in medical surgery.

In addition to advancements in medical tools and technologies, anatomical dissection had a profound impact on medical knowledge, particularly in respect to internal human anatomy and physiology. Although human dissection had been intermittently practiced in Europe since the thirteenth century (Brenna 2021), dissection and anatomization did not become an accepted practice within the American medical community until at least after the Civil War, when individual states passed laws regulating dissection as a branch of medical science (Richardson 2001). During the eighteenth century, only the bodies of convicted criminals could be legally used for medical research. Dissection was often framed as a further punitive measure for committing a crime, thus securing the link between criminality and the loss of bodily rights after death (Nystrom et al. 2017). Students and faculty at medical schools were often complicit in illegally taking recently deceased, marginalized individuals from graves (Highet 2005; Shultz 2005). Beginning in the late 1800s, states passed anatomy acts that made unclaimed bodies available to medical schools and hospitals for teaching and research (Devine 2016).

Archaeologists have shown how dissection and anatomization were foundational to the development of professional medicine during the nineteenth century (Hodge et al. 2017; Nystrom 2014, 2017). In Massachusetts, the Harvard Anatomical Society was formed in 1771 and the Harvard Medical School in 1782 (Hodge 2013). At Harvard University, Holden Chapel operated as a lecture hall devoted to anatomical and science education until 1862 (Hodge 2013: 126). Archaeological excavations of a dry well at Holden produced 3,316 fragments of animal remains, human bones, architectural remains, glassware, ceramics, architectural debris, and unknown substances (Hodge 2013: 128; Hodge et al. 2017). Multiple human bones evidenced dissection techniques, such as transverse cuts through femurs and tibias. Some elements may have exhibited surgical cuts for amputations. Many of these individuals were likely "unclaimed" at death—the indigent, homeless, or minoritized social groups that were unable to secure a proper burial. (The 1831 Anatomy Act of Massachusetts allowed medical schools to acquire unclaimed bodies of the destitute, insane, ill, and formerly imprisoned.) Similar research at the Medical College of Georgia uncovered over 10,000 human bones in the basement of the building (Blakely and Harrington 1997: 107). Dissection was illegal in Georgia until 1887 and, as at many other teaching colleges, individual bodies were procured illegally. Following medical dissection, bodies were unceremoniously disposed of in medical waste pits, along with other objects such as bottles, medical implements, clothing items, and animal bones (Blakely and Harrington 1997: 108).

Physicians' use of unclaimed bodies for anatomical science reified existing structural social and legal inequalities (Muller et al. 2017). The different "postmortem interventions" (Crossland 2009) to which people were subjected tended to vary according to their social identities. "The bodies of elites and bourgeoisie were considered appropriate *subjects* for autopsy,[2] while the bodies of the poor and disenfranchised were *objects* for dissection" (Novak 2017: 88). Medical expertise was created through the power-laden relationships between dead individuals and anatomists. Bodies used for dissection were often acquired from enslaved and free Black cemeteries, potter's fields for unknown and indigent people, and graveyards associated with jails and almshouses (Chapman and Kostro 2017; Richardson

---

2 *Autopsy* refers to scientific investigations of an individual cause of death, not dissection for the purpose of promoting medical training and knowledge. Autopsies were exceptional and rarely performed in the eighteenth and nineteenth centuries.

2001). By the 1830s, Black bodies were regularly used for medical experimentation (including dissection), a practice that continued during the postbellum period (Halperin 2007; Savitt 1982). Persons dissected in the name of medical science were marginalized members of society during life, remained nameless in death, and have largely been forgotten by subsequent generations (Blakely and Harrington 1997; Chapman and Kostro 2017; Nystrom 2014, 2017; Werner and Novak 2010).

Bioarchaeological research has explored the ways medical scientists exploited definitions of personhood via the performative nature of body acquisition and dissection, specimen preparation, the use of body parts in educational lectures, and the disposal of bodies after their medical "use value" expired (Hodge 2013). The bodies of dissected individuals represented multiple meanings throughout the course of dissection: illegal contraband, scientific subjects, and ultimately medical waste (Novak 2017). This work contributes to a burgeoning critique in the broader social sciences regarding the endemic violence within the discipline of American medicine. As scholars in related fields have demonstrated, scientists' nonvoluntary, dangerous, and exploitative experimentation on Black and other minoritized bodies has been documented since the eighteenth century (for a comprehensive review and case studies, see Savitt 1982 and Washington 2006). Archaeological research on dissection, anatomization, and other partible practices foregrounds the importance of studying the violent foundations of medical practice and knowledge making, the legacies of racist epistemologies in contemporary clinical practice, and the ethical requirements that guide the study of marginalized groups in bioarchaeological research (Zuckerman, Kamnikar, and Mathena 2014).

Medical Education: Medical Schools, Training, and Licensing

In addition to new medical technologies and educational programs, official training and licensing programs developed by medical associations and enforced by state and federal legislators during the eighteenth through twentieth centuries had a profound impact on the professional medical field. Organizations such as the AMA would be instrumental in consolidating the power and authority of physicians—a halting process that predated the AMA's founding in the mid-nineteenth century. Indeed, from the 1760s, educated doctors attempted to create a cohesive and exclusive field of medicine that only admitted professionally trained physicians. These attempts were thwarted by state legislatures that voted to do away with state licensing entirely, along with rural and urban populaces that were skeptical of professional medicine (Starr 2017: 31).

During the American colonial period, few practicing physicians received formal training in the form of university education. A small number of doctors were trained at universities in England, Scotland, or France, while a minority of New England physicians graduated from Harvard College (Starr 2017). Most medical practitioners gained experience and training via three practical routes: an apprenticeship with a local practitioner, a proprietary school at which students received training from the physician who owned and operated the medical college, or through a university where students received a combination of didactic and clinical training (Beck 2004: 2139). Medical schools and independent practitioners taught an array of theories and practices, from scientific medicine to osteopathy, homeopathy, herbalism, hydrotherapy, and physio-medical and Thomsonian medicine (Whorton 2004). As Shryock notes, "We now speak customarily of the medical profession as if there were only one; meaning, of course, the physician" (Shryock 1936). But physicians constituted just one arm of medicine; nurses, midwives, herbalists, pharmacists, surgeons, and itinerant healers were also significant medical providers in their communities. It was also common for medical practitioners, including doctors, to perform other trades besides medicine (Starr 2017: 39). A 1773 advertisement for a midwife stated that she cured "ringworms, scald heads, piles, and worms" and made "dresses and bonnets in the latest fashion" (Starr 2017: 39).

In the 1830s and 1840s, a renewed national sense of individualism and anti-professionalism hindered physicians' attempts to implement standardized training and licensing as requirements for practice (Shortt 1983). But by the mid- to late nineteenth century, politicians' interest in implementing state and federal licensing regulations, scientific developments in diagnosing procedures in medicine, and vaccination programs increased the credibility of physicians among the general public (Duffy 1993; Haller 1981). By 1860, the AMA had a large, robust membership capable of lobbying state legislatures to implement (or re-implement) medical licensing laws. In 1867, medical societies began instituting licensing reforms and the US government started sponsoring research for infectious diseases (Devine 2016: 153). Throughout the latter half of the 1800s, the AMA advocated for the standardization of medical training, including implementing standard university curriculums and mandatory, applied training programs. These attempts were met with resistance by federal lawmakers, in part due to political traditions in the United States that dissuaded national government oversight of private professions (Beck 2004: 2139). By the early 1900s, the AMA had implemented mandatory educational and licensing requirements for all practicing physicians. Members of the AMA also became increasingly convinced of the effectiveness of scientific medical practice. The organization argued that medical students and practicing physicians should apply the scientific method and be actively engaged in laboratory experimentation and hands-on care throughout their careers (Beck 2004: 2139; Rothstein 1987).

In 1904, the AMA created the Council on Medical Education (CME) to develop standards in medical training and education and to implement a standard medical curriculum (Rothstein 1987). In 1908, the CME contracted with the Carnegie Foundation for the Advancement of Education to assess the state of medical training in the United States. An independent researcher, Abraham Flexner, was tasked with visiting 155 medical schools across the country (Beck 2004). In 1910, the results of Flexner's study, aptly named the "Flexner Report," were released (Cooke et al. 2006; Flexner 1925). Flexner demonstrated that there were vast differences in resources (primarily clinical and laboratory spaces) and educators between medical schools. His proposed solution was to reroute funding to a few, exceptional programs and guarantee state government oversight of medical training (Beck 2004). He also stressed that medical education should emphasize learning the scientific method and acquiring clinical experience in academic hospitals (Barr 2010: 36; Cooke et al. 2006). Flexner recommended that students undergo a premedical training program prior to entering medical school, which secured student admissions among a few, elite medical schools.

The Flexner Report is considered one of the most impactful undertakings in American medicine and has had lasting administrative, financial, and practical consequences for both physicians and patients in the United States. Flexner advised defunding and/or closing schools and programs that taught "non-conformist" approaches in medicine. These included chiropractic medicine, osteopathy, and homeopathy (Stahnisch and Verhoef 2012: 2), which Flexner called "quackery" and "charlatanism." Flexner's report also severely constrained the role of Black doctors within the medical community by arguing that these doctors' practices were to be "limited to [their] own race" (Sullivan and Suez Mittman 2010: 248). Black doctors were to be excluded from participating in medical research and were to "maintain the principles of hygiene, sanitation, and civilization" among members of Black communities (Sullivan and Suez Mittman 2010: 248). The Flexner Report also recommended that four of six historically Black colleges be closed, including Leonard Medical School, which was the largest Black medical school (Williams et al. 2021). The report facilitated admissions policies and educational standards that were inaccessible to Black students, therefore limiting the role and presence of Black doctors in American medical practice (Beck 2004; Sullivan and Suez Mittman 2010: 247). Premedical (premed) education requirements, along with the financial inaccessibility of medical school, created a climate of professional elitism that dissuaded racialized minorities and economically disadvantaged students from pursuing careers in medicine (Harley 2006; Steinecke and Terrell 2010). The report had lasting impacts on professional medicine; in 1950, students from underrepresented minority backgrounds made up only 1 percent of graduating classes from all US medical schools (Barr 2010: 133).

Household and Community-Based Medicine

Education and licensing programs implemented by the AMA and state legislatures, largely resulting from the Flexner Report, created a field of medical practice that excluded participation by ethnic and racial minorities. Expensive medical schools and training programs meant that medical education and licensing were accessible only to white, middle- to upper-class men. In addition, in 1847 the AMA fixed the cost of certain medical services, which rendered most medical procedures and ethical (prescription) medications unaffordable to lower-income households. Disparities created by unequal access to professional medical care and to medical training programs encouraged members of marginalized and minoritized social groups to seek care via alternative means. In addition to the structural and economic restraints faced by Black communities, immigrants, impoverished communities, and gendered minorities, many people avoided professionally educated and trained doctors for personal reasons. These included doctors' use of radical and invasive treatments on their patients, centuries of discriminatory and racist scientific theories of medicine and the body, and citizens' pervasive distrust of medical elitism. The majority of the American population from the colonial period until the post–World War

I era relied on some form of community or home care that fell outside the purview of professional medicine (Johnston 2004; Whorton 2004).

Despite institutional and government changes to the professional medical field during the nineteenth and twentieth centuries, access to professional medical care remained uneven. Rural populations were frequently unable to physically access physicians and clinics (Starr 2017), and racism and gender discrimination pervaded the professional medical field to such an extent that African Americans, immigrants, women, and other marginalized populations were largely excluded from or distrustful of professional care (Gamble 1993, 1997; Institute of Medicine [US] Committee on Understanding and Eliminating Racial and Ethnic Disparities in Health Care 2002).

As the historical and archaeological case studies in this chapter demonstrate, alternative healing systems were not merely markers of patient noncompliance or ignorance. These systems of healing and preventative care were developed by communities who perceived a need for alternative methods of care. Black Americans, Indigenous people, women, and other marginalized social groups also relied on diverse methods that did not ontologically divorce bodily health from spiritual, mental, and community well-being. Healing practices reflected these varying epistemological frameworks of disease and medicine; health officials' opinions of what constituted "good care" often deviated from the medical practices performed within professional medicine. Finally, "alternative" therapies comprise a significant number of nonbiomedical healing practices, both in the past and in the present. Today, alternative practices, or CAM, are an integral part of the American medical landscape, especially for marginalized and minoritized communities.

Women's Health and Reproductive Care

Despite some scholars' tendencies to view the American healthcare system as a relatively homogeneous and monolithic system, the medical landscape in the United States has been diverse and marked by resistance to the professional care sector (Porter 2003; Shryock 1936). During the eighteenth and nineteenth centuries, domestic medicine (or "irregular" medicine as it is sometimes called) and professional medicine comprised parallel sectors of the healthcare field (Starr 2017: 32). Nonprofessional medicine has historically been performed in the domestic sphere, predominately by women, who were trained by family members, members of their own community, or to a lesser extent, in professional medical schools. Historical archaeologists have shown how communities who were excluded from accessing professional care, or who were distrustful of the professional medical community, created networks of healthcare and support that fell outside the purview of medical organizations and trained physicians' oversight.

Archaeologies of women's health and healthcare, in particular, have largely focused on reproductive agency and self-care, how systems of power shaped patterns of access to reproductive care, and intersectional approaches that show how race, gender, and class affected experiences of reproduction (Jenkins 2020). Archaeologists have addressed women's experiences as mothers and their reproductive and sexual health, especially in regard to contraception, abortion, and childbirth (Barnes 2021; Jenkins 2020; Wilkie 2003). They have critiqued the tendency to focus narrowly on women's reproductive health, advocating for a broader, more inclusive approach that views sexual and reproductive health as one of many interlocking facets of women's "daily health lives" (Morton 2013: 4). Medical devices commonly found in archaeological contexts, such as douches and syringes, may have been used as contraceptive tools, but they must also be interpreted within a broader framework of women's agency, gendered practices, and medical meaning making (Morton 2013: 5). For example, vaginal douching can be interpreted as a complex practice involving self-diagnosis and self-treatment, incorporating strategic decisions regarding product availability, perceived effectiveness, and interpretations of "normal" health (Morton 2013).

Women's health realities were drawn along gendered and racialized lines. A university education was one route by which white women could enter the professional medical field. By the mid-nineteenth century, white (often middle-class) women were sometimes allowed entry into medical schools (Morantz-Sanchez 2005: 64). Nevertheless, by 1893, only 37 of 165 medical training programs had admitted women (Morantz-Sanchez 2005). Women's medical colleges, such as the Women's Medical College of New York, were established in response to these exclusionary practices. Still, many women physicians nonetheless argued that coeducation was important and felt "very strongly the advantage of admission to the large organized system of public instruction already existing for men" (Morantz-Sanchez 2005: 66), claiming the benefits that coeducation and collegiality could offer. Postgraduation, women living in the mid- to late nineteenth century encountered success in private practice, working in hospitals, or teaching in medical institutions. Women physicians found ready acceptance within immigrant communities in urban areas and were often requested by female patients (Morantz-Sanchez 2005: 151).

During the mid-nineteenth century, white middle-class women adopted more participatory roles in health reform movements, which came to be known as the "health crusades" (Morantz 1977: 496). Women reformers, including Mary Gove Nichols, Rachel Brooks Gleason, and Lydia Folger Fowler, came from middle-class Northeastern families (Morantz-Sanchez 2005: 33). These reformers eschewed outdated notions that couched femininity in terms of sickness and weakness. Instead, they adopted Enlightenment ideals of wellness and physical strength, claiming that good health was a fundamental human right for both men and women and that good health was the key to the modern woman's improved status (Morantz-Sanchez 2005). Women's health reformers recognized that male physicians and their attendant practices were often sexist and harmed women's health, especially in the realms of gynecology and childbirth. Rather than rely on the ineffectual and "irreparably injurious" treatments offered by male physicians, women encouraged each other to become educated and create communities of mutual support (Morantz 1977: 495). Homeopathic journals were widely popular with literate women, referencing the importance of family planning, preventative medicine, and healthy lifestyles to modern women. Archaeological excavations at the Talbot County Women's Club property in Easton, Maryland, uncovered an advertising booklet for abortion pills, including Chichester's booklet, along with a collection of young children's toys. The artifacts were associated with a lower-middle-class household in the early twentieth century. Their presence indicates that women at the residence managed their own reproductive health and participated in the new ideology of scientific motherhood (Jenkins 2020: 595). The advertisement and toys indicate the "complex decisions that women had to make about having or not having children and how to raise those that they did have" (Jenkins 2020: 595).

Experiences related to reproductive health and education for Black women during the nineteenth and early twentieth centuries differed significantly from middle-class white women's experiences. Intergenerational poverty and poor living conditions negatively affected Black women's health and contributed to low fertility rates (Roberts 2017). Life expectancy was also low (mid-thirties) while infant mortality and morbidity rates were higher than those of their white counterparts. Black women's organizations tried to open their own medical clinics, but these efforts were largely unsuccessful because of a lack of public support and funding (Roberts 2017: 87). Intersectional approaches to archaeological and historical records demonstrate how race, class, gender, and sexuality influenced Black women's health and agency throughout their lives (Jenkins 2020). Archaeologists demonstrate how Black women were kept away from professional medicine via segregation from medical clinics, exclusion from the birth control movement, and a distrust of white doctors (Jenkins 2020).

Using artifacts recovered from the Hollywood Plantation in Drew County, Arkansas, Barnes (2021: 10) uses an intersectional lens to "examine the ways that women were/are racialized and deemed less than full persons through what Faye Ginsburg and Rayna Rapp (1995) term 'stratified reproduction.'" Barnes uses the concept of stratified reproduction to refer to the power relations that shape access to or limit reproductive choices. Instead of solely focusing on health-related objects, such as medicine bottles, Barnes expands the repertoire of reproduction-related material items to include ceramics, doll parts, and grave markers. If reproductive oppression permeates all aspects of women's lived experiences, the material correlates to these experiences should be similarly ubiquitous in the archaeological record. For example, safety pins found at the Hollywood Plantation may have been used to alter women's clothing during pregnancy or to fasten children's diapers (Barnes 2021: 14). Stone and wooden grave markers are material markers of maternal loss and the racialized dehumanization of Black women. At the plantation, Kittie Ann Prosper worked as a laundress, cook, domestic, and nursemaid, doing the majority of the "motherwork" for her own family and for the owners of the plantation, the Taylors. Children's toys that were recovered archaeologically show the intimate relationship that Prosper had with the Taylor children as a primary caregiver who still inhabited a separate part of the household (Barnes 2021: 25). Historical archaeologies of reproductive violence contextualize forms of structural anti-Blackness in the present by uncovering the historical roots of reproductive inequality (Barnes 2021: 28). Today, Black women are more likely to die in childbirth than their white counterparts, and they suffer from significantly higher rates of pregnancy-related morbidities (Taylor 2020). Poor health outcomes among Black women cannot be solely attributed to unequal access to care or poverty but are directly related to structural racism and historical systems of oppression (Taylor 2020: 506).

In the southern and eastern United States, African American midwives provided care to Black women. Midwives assisted women in pregnancy, delivered babies, and gave important information to their patients regarding abortion and contraception (Jenkins 2020; Wilkie 2003). Archaeological material recovered from the Alabama household of a Black midwife, Lucrecia Perryman, includes animal remains, medicine bottles, foods, and tools that can be used to interpret the embodied experiences of pregnancy and birth (Wilkie 2003). As Wilkie (2003) argues, African American midwives did not distinguish between spiritual and bodily health and often integrated care practices from different cultural traditions, including those rooted in African philosophies, Enlightenment theories of hygiene and medicine, and magical practices shared with European-American healers. For example, botanical medicines used across ethnomedical traditions for abortifacients and birth control included ginger, okra, and castor oil (Wilkie 2013). Ritual materials that served to protect parents and infants have been found archaeologically; pierced coins, hand amulets, and beads were likely used to offer magical protection (Wilkie 2013).

Menstruation, sex, gestation, and childbirth are experienced in non-universal ways that entail distinct communities of practice. As such, these embodied experiences leave behind a rich and diverse record of material practices. Archaeologists must carefully contextualize botanical, faunal, and material assemblages with robust ethnohistorical and ethnographic sources in order to capture the full range of healing practices in the past.

Community-Based Healthcare Systems

Historical archaeological research has demonstrated a) the poor health outcomes historically suffered by Black communities in the Americas; b) the extent to which Black communities, households, and individual patients were excluded from accessing professional care; and c) the ways in which Black communities created institutions and networks of care within their own communities as a response to structural racism. Archaeological research on health and healthcare patterns among African American populations in Washington, DC, touches upon all three of these key themes. Using historical and archaeological sources, Dunnavant (2017) argues that social and political circumstances during the Reconstruction era negatively impacted the health outcomes of African Americans. Formerly enslaved populations were vulnerable to smallpox, cholera, tuberculosis, and fevers, while urbanization and poverty compounded the effects of disease outbreaks (Dunnavant 2017: 115). Health disparities were related to overall quality of life and poor living conditions, but also likely resulted from unequal access to professional care. Dunnavant's study pairs bioarchaeological data from the Mount Pleasant Plains Cemetery with demographic data from municipal death records to investigate health outcomes among Black communities in Washington, DC, and patterns of access to end-of-life care. Bioarchaeological analyses of individuals from the Mount Pleasant Plains Cemetery demonstrate that access to end-of-life care among African Americans buried at the cemetery was contingent upon gender and employment. Unemployed Black women were particularly vulnerable populations, with the least access to professional care at the end of their lives.

During the Civil War and Reconstruction period, public hospitals were reserved for those who could not afford to see a doctor at home or who did not have a family to care for them. Hospitals did not function as clinical care institutions like they do today but were affiliated with other charitable organizations such as almshouses and asylums (Risse 2016). Freedmen's hospitals cared for Black individuals and were known for being particularly underfunded and understaffed. As a response to inadequate healthcare services, African Americans organized alternative methods of healthcare (Dunnavant 2017: 126). Mount Pleasant Plains Cemetery (opened in 1870) was founded by the Free Young Men's Benevolent Association to serve African Americans who were denied burial in white cemeteries in Washington, DC. This mutual-aid society also provided healthcare services to members in need, especially families who were affected by sickness or death.

In addition to aid societies, Black churches and religious communities have a long history of addressing the health needs of Black communities (Chatters et al. 1998; Taylor et al. 2000, 2004). Archaeological research conducted at the Wayman African Methodist Episcopal Church in Bloomington, Illinois, underscores the importance of religious organizations in providing health services to Black congregations (Cabak et al. 1995). Black churches fulfilled multiple roles within their communities: they were places for spiritual and educational guidance and spaces that provided care for sick and suffering members (Cabak et al. 1995: 357). Archaeological excavations at the Wayman African Methodist Episcopal Church focused on its outbuildings and rear yard. Predominately food-related items were found, suggesting that community meals were an important function of the church. Glass medicine bottles and healthcare equipment constituted a large percentage of the personal items, also suggesting that the church provided healthcare services to the congregation and community. Most of the medicine bottles were prescription instead of patent medicine. The prescription medicines could have been purchased directly from a pharmacy. Or, as the authors tentatively suggest, they may have been provided by Dr. Gray Covington, the only Black physician in Bloomington, whose office was located near the church. The authors argue that the presence of healthcare-related artifacts represents the African American community's reaction to medical care inequality and poorer health outcomes through "self-help" programs (Cabak et al. 1995).

Community-based healthcare strategies were not exclusive to Black communities in the United States. They were also fundamental to other racialized and economically disadvantaged communities that could not access physician care or were distrustful of trained and licensed doctors. In addition to using ineffective and physically traumatic treatments, licensed physicians were often reluctant to care for poor or marginalized people (Rosenberg 2003). As a result, immigrant neighborhoods, racialized minority groups, and other marginalized groups participated in informal economies of care at both the household and community scale. Archaeological research at Chinese railroad workers' sites in California, Idaho, Montana, Texas, Utah, and Nevada demonstrates the importance of patent medicines and Chinese medicines for immigrant communities (Heffner 2013, 2015). In the western United States, Chinese railroad workers were organized into isolated work camps and would not have had access to formally trained Chinese doctors, who resided in urban Chinatowns (Heffner 2015). As Voss (2018) notes, historical records indicating the exploitative living and working conditions of workers and artifactual evidence from railroad sites suggest that workers had little choice regarding goods, services, and foods. Thus, railroad workers relied on informal systems of medicine and self-treated with plants, animals, teas, and nonprescription medicines. Healthcare-related objects from railroad workers' sites include homeopathic medicine vials, Chinese medicine vials, opium-smoking paraphernalia, patent medicine bottles, teacups, and floral and faunal remains (Heffner 2013, 2015).

Archaeological research in Five Points, New York, also illustrates the importance of community-based care by showing how Irish American families mitigated the threats of disease in response to recurring cholera epidemics and the deleterious health effects of unsanitary living conditions (Bonasera and Raymer 2001). Archaeological findings at Five Points show that because physicians in New York were expensive and inaccessible to most working-class families, Five Points residents were unlikely to have relied on visiting doctors to cure their illnesses. Dispensaries, charitable hospitals, and apothecaries were the most affordable and accessible sources of medicine for immigrant, working-class, and low-income families in the Five Points neighborhood. The New York Dispensary was the only dispensary in the Sixth Ward in the 1860s, and it claimed to have treated over 50,000 sick poor on an annual basis (Bonasera and Raymer 2001). A children's hospital at the Five Points House of Industry operated in the 1880s and wrote over 3,000 prescriptions in 1884. In addition, many apothecaries operating in the neighborhood provided a convenient source of patent and ethical medicines. Proprietary medicines could be purchased directly by consumers from retailers; these included popular, nationally marketed products, as well as medicines that were only produced in New York. An analysis of proprietary medicine bottles from Five Points suggests that residents were interested in treating the symptoms of rheumatism, soreness, strains, burns, "feminine disorders," colic, venereal diseases, and blood diseases (Bonasera and Raymer 2001: 51). Five Points residents also used herbal remedies, as evidenced by an archaeobotanical assemblage that included mint, mustard, cherry, raspberry/blackberry, elderberry, strawberry, boneset, dock, pokeweed, jimsonweed, and wormseed. All these plants were commonly used in nineteenth-century home remedies (Bonasera and Raymer 2001: 56). In sum, Five Points residents developed a complex system of healthcare that included home remedies, such as plants, proprietary medicines, and ethical medicines. In the absence of citywide sanitation measures and access to licensed physicians, residents of Block 160 and other tenements developed methods of self-care to mitigate the deleterious health conditions of nineteenth-century New York (Bonasera and Raymer 2001: 62).

Archaeological research in other Irish American communities demonstrates similar patterns of access to professional medical care. Brighton (2005: 250) notes that self-medication was important to Irish immigrant communities in New York, since Irish immigrants typically could not afford physician expenses, or they were discriminated against by professional doctors. Alienation from formal healthcare services precipitated complex networks of informal self-care regimes, which relied on household knowledge systems and administration of proprietary drugs (Brighton 2005). Archaeological research at Sorinsville, a predominately Irish Catholic community in South Bend, Indiana during the 1850s and 1860s, shows how residents navigated the daily social and political complexities of transnational identity politics and discrimination. Sixteen medicine bottles were recovered from excavations at the Fogarty family house lot, which was occupied from the 1860s until the early twentieth century (Rotman

2010). The majority of the bottles (thirteen) represented patent and proprietary medicines; only a single bottle represented an ethical, or doctor-prescribed, medicine (Rotman 2010: 123). Although the family had access to St. Joseph's Hospital, founded by a convent and likely to receive Irish Catholic patients, Rotman argues that the hospital's history as an institution for convicts and the poor would have made it undesirable. Instead of seeking care from physicians or hospitals, self-treatment would have been a manageable option, and one that gave family members control over their own treatments.

Holistic Healing and Pluralistic Medicinal Traditions

Women, Black Americans, immigrant communities, and other marginalized people were often wary of, or excluded from, accessing professional medical care; as a result, they often participated in alternative (or homeopathic) models of healthcare. Other practitioners of alternative medicine were discontented with the invasive and costly treatments offered by trained and licensed physicians. Today, alternative medicine commonly typically falls under the category of CAM. Functional definitions of CAM comprise all practices not derived from Western biomedicine. These include various ethnic traditions, practices such as reflexology and herbal medicine, and approaches whose origins do not lie in Western scientific theory (Thorne et al. 2002). Other definitions of CAM include "health systems, modalities, practices and their accompanying theories and beliefs that are not intrinsic to the politically dominant health system of a particular society or culture in a given historical period" (Ning 2013: 136). CAM practices are often derived from ideological factors, such as holism, vitalism, spirituality, and natural healing (Ning 2013).

While CAM is a contemporary term used to describe alternative medical systems in the present, alternative models of healing have a long history in the United States (Whorton 2004). I use the term *alternative medicine* to refer to therapeutic practices that were not supported by and taught by the professional medical field (as part of orthodox practice) and were not grounded in scientific theories of medicine. Alternative or "nonorthodox" healing systems in the late seventeenth through twentieth centuries were incredibly diverse and included herbal and plant-based medicine, homeopathy, and astrology, to name a few (Whorton 2004). Self-treatment and alternative medical practices in the nineteenth century coincided with a surge in patent medicine production and advertising, which foregrounded the significance of self-medication and self-care. Common alternative practices included spirituality and spiritual healing, natural cures, hydropathy, and holism. As the archaeological studies in this chapter demonstrate, alternative therapies were not rooted in a single, overarching political or ideological system, but developed out of myriad political and social circumstances. Pragmatic reasons for turning to alternative medicine may include distrust in the professional medical field, concerns about conventional treatments, the perceived higher effectiveness of alternative therapies, and patients' desire to actively participate in self-care regimes, particularly in respect to managing chronic conditions (Thorne et al. 2002). By the mid- to late 1800s, Euro-American patients increasingly sought less dangerous and more ameliorative healing methods than those offered by the professional medical community, often turning to alternative therapies and herbal medicines, which they deemed more "natural" and less physically invasive. "Natural" healthcare strategies involved herbal treatments, recourse to spiritual means for treating illness, and diverse hydrotherapeutic measures.

Spiritual and herbal healing practices have a long history in the United States and are practiced today among both Native and non-Native communities. Ethnomedical traditions of Native North American tribes are grounded in long-standing relationships with the land and exhibit an intimate understanding of floral and faunal populations (Cohen 1998; Portman and Garrett 2006). Ethnomedical traditions do not adopt physicalist and functionalist accounts of the body and disease, but rather view bodily health as the outcome of a nexus of spiritual, physical, and community well-being (Hutchinson 2022). Global processes, including European colonialism, plantation slavery and the transatlantic slave trade, and migrations from Asian countries to the United States hastened the development of new, pluralistic medicinal innovations and practices. Native American ethnobotanical healing customs were of considerable interest to early European colonial populations (Vogel 1990). The integration of Native American, African, and Euro-American ethnobotanical healing practices resulted in diverse, pluralistic medicinal systems in America from the seventeenth through twentieth centuries. Historical and archaeological research communities in North America demonstrate how social interactions between cultural groups spurred diverse, "creolized" ethnobotanical healing practices (Mrozowski et al. 2008). For example, Iroquois use of blue lobelia (*Lobelia siphilitica*) as a remedy for syphilis was later adopted by Euro-Americans for the same purpose. It was also used as an expectorant, emetic, and diuretic in Thomsonian medicine (Vogel 1990: 48). Cadwallader Colden (1688–1776), a physician and botanist, commented on the usefulness of "Indian pokeroot" (*Phytolacca decandra* L.) as a cure for cancer based on knowledge that he acquired from Mohawks (Vogel 1990: 49). Thomas Ashe, writing in 1682, noted the healing practices of Carolina Native people, who used "incantations" and plant-based medicines (Vogel 1990). Some plants used in Native practices, such as snakeroot and sassafras, appear in multiple European accounts as popular herbal remedies for everything from fevers to "pleurisy" (Vogel 1990).

Archaeological research at the Sandy Site in Roanoke, Virginia, recovered several plants with medicinal qualities dating to the Late Woodland period (AD 900–1607) (Vanderwarker and Stanyard 2009). The site was a short-term seasonal encampment or kill and butcher site. The macrobotanical assemblage includes nutritionally and medicinally significant plant taxa, which may have functioned as a kind of "first aid kit" (Vanderwarker and Stanyard 2009: 145). The most prevalent plant in the assemblage with medicinal qualities was bearsfoot (*Polymnia uvedalia*), which is used in poultices and can be imbibed as a laxative and stimulant. Holly seeds (*Ilex vomitoria*) may be used as an emetic, while wax myrtle (*Myrica* sp.) is a widely documented plant for treating ulcers, diarrhea, dysentery, jaundice, and uterine bleeding. Bedstraw (*Galium* sp.) may have been prepared as a tea (Vanderwarker and Stanyard 2009: 135).

Archaeological excavations at Thomas Jefferson's plantation in Rich Neck, Virginia, revealed a similarly complex range of plant resources. By conducting a temporal analysis of plant procurement and use through time at the site, then comparing these results to inventory records from Rich Neck, the authors conclude that social organization was a key factor in bringing diverse knowledge and resources to members of the household (Mrozowski et al. 2008: 708). They connect household lifecycles and household strategies to medicinal plant use and foodways. Enslaved people at Rich Neck developed foodways and medicinal systems that incorporated European, African, and Native American practices and knowledge systems (Mrozowski et al. 2008). Honey locust (*Gleditsia triacanthos* L.) and black walnut (*Juglans nigra*) were prevalent in the assemblage as a whole. Both species have documented medicinal and nutritional uses by the Cherokee, Delaware, Rappahannock, Creek, and Fox (Mrozowski et al. 2008: 712). Households at Rich Neck may have utilized the plants as sweeteners, skin ointments, and teas.

Archaeologists also challenge scholars to critically reflect on how they interpret floral and faunal remains and health-related objects from archaeological contexts. This work challenges presentist ontologies of biomedicine by showing how cultural groups often do not distinguish between food and medicine; nor do they draw definitive distinctions between the health of the physical, spiritual, and social communal bodies. Paleoethnobotanical studies, in particular, have broadened our understanding of how provisioned, gardened/produced, and procured plants met important nutritional, medicinal, and psychological needs for Native American and Black communities (Mrozowski et al. 2008). Mrozowski and colleagues (2008: 700) develop a "well-being" approach to investigate how enslaved people used plants in the context of violence, racism, and economic and biological deprivation to meet culturally defined standards of emotional and physical health. In their analysis of macrobotanical remains from the eighteenth-century Rich Neck Plantation in Virginia, they demonstrate how changes in plant species ubiquity from different temporal contexts indicate shifting plantation provisioning systems, alterations in household subsistence strategies, and changes in healthcare strategies through time. Instead of attempting to differentiate between different functional qualities of plants from Rich Neck (in other words, as either food or medicine), the authors instead show how different plant species may have been used to meet the spiritual, nutritional, and psychosocial health needs of the community.

My archaeological research at a former rural hospital in St. Croix, US Virgin Islands, demonstrates how European colonialism and plantation slavery shaped cosmopolitan medical systems (Reifschneider 2018; Reifschneider and Bardolph 2020). This work also mobilizes Mrozowski et al.'s (2008) concept of "well-being" to show how foods and local plants contributed to the health of enslaved people. While St. Croix was administered by the Danish crown from the eighteenth century until 1917, the island's healthcare system merged policies, practices, and medical theories from the United States, Denmark, and enslaved African communities to address the island's unique healthcare needs. Many of the practicing physicians in the Virgin Islands were trained in US medical programs and/or were American by birth. Doctors also adhered to medical theories developed in the United States, while pharmacies on St. Croix were required by Danish law to import only compounding agents from the United States (Reifschneider 2019). Following the abolition of the slave trade in 1803, the Danish crown established a centralized healthcare system to oversee the health of both white colonial and Black enslaved populations in their Caribbean holdings, to include St. Croix, St. John, and St. Thomas (Jen-

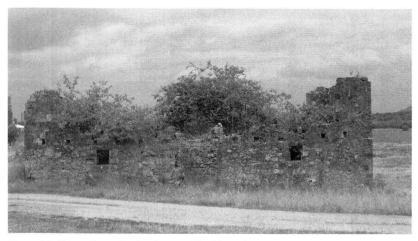

Figure 2.3. Estate Cane Garden hospital building, facing south.

sen 2012). Demographic records from churches and public hospitals indicate that enslaved people suffered from numerous health conditions, such as infectious diseases like intermittent fevers (malaria and yellow fever), nutritional diseases, and work-related trauma (Jensen 2012). European-trained physicians from England, America, and Scotland were tasked with attending to enslaved Black, free Black, and white patients.

Research at the former plantation hospital of Estate Cane Garden demonstrates how the colonial healthcare system intersected with local care practices at plantation hospitals (Figure 2.3) (Reifschneider 2018). Danish medical records indicate that Scottish-born physician Dr. Christopher Johnson, who was trained at Yale Medical School, attended the plantation, although an enslaved nurse performed daily care at the hospital. Archaeological investigations of the Estate Cane Garden hospital indicate that allopathic treatments, such as venesection, cupping, and apothecary medicines, were not common there (Reifschneider 2018). Instead, faunal and macrobotanical evidence suggests that plantation nurses relied on herbal treatments and diverse foods to care for their patients (Reifschneider and Bardolph 2020). This work complicates archaeological classification systems that often obscure the dynamic origins and use lives of medicinal resources and demonstrates the importance of examining plant and animal residues as active, dynamic agents in healthcare regimens.

Spiritual Healing and the Return to Nature

Spiritual healing practices have a long history in Europe and its colonies and post-colonies. For example, in Britain and Denmark during the eighteenth century, most of the population relied on folk healers who utilized aspects of magic and ritual in their healing cures (Bonderup et al. 2001). Scientific medical practitioners remained a small contingent of the healing community, and for most, healing involved treating the physical and spiritual corpus. From the seventeenth through early twentieth centuries, bodily ontologies and healing practices were underscored by spiritual concerns. Adherents of spiritual healing claimed that diverse forms of spirituality guided one's relationship to the natural world and fundamentally altered one's bodily health (Bonderup et al. 2001).

In early colonial period America, Protestant cultures held that standards of health and medical misfortunes had spiritual origins. Both lay doctors and patients recognized disease as a sign of God's displeasure and a warning to those who were immoral. As Loren (2013: 153) notes, the moral soul and physical body were inseparable, and physical illness was a result of a corrupt soul. Medical afflictions were attributed to the will of God as punishment for sins; patients were encouraged to reflect upon their moral inadequacies and learn the lessons of God through recovery. Only church clergy could ameliorate the spiritual causes of disease, while physicians could work in conjunction with clergy to alleviate the physical symptoms of illness.

As Loren (2013, 2015, 2016) argues, bodily comportment and sartorial presentation were also paramount in securing one's moral and hence physical health. Loren's archaeological and archival research in Massachusetts at colonial Harvard demonstrates how anxieties regarding the body shaped sartorial conventions and how Puritan values were mobilized to protect the moral and physical health of students and colonized Native Americans. Seventeenth-century New Englanders were subject to an onslaught of infectious diseases: whipworm, roundworm, malaria, smallpox, and yellow fever (Loren 2013). Remains of pharmaceutical bottles, macrobotanical remains, clothing items, and smoking pipes suggest a rich healing history at Harvard. Coin charms were used on the body to protect against sin and illness, while smoking tobacco was thought to be an efficient curative for diseases such as cancer and respiratory illness. Macrobotanical remains found in Loren's investigations included henbane and thorn apple. Both plants can be toxic, but when prepared and used carefully, they can treat the symptoms of respiratory illness (Loren 2013). Loren's research demonstrates how Puritan anxieties concerning bodily and spiritual decline shaped the lived experiences and material lives of the Harvard community.

The early nineteenth century saw a return to Evangelicalism and a renewed interest in the relationship between the human body, God, and health. Reformers advocated for a return to the natural world, thus reaching a higher level of spirituality and well-being. During the nineteenth century, Americans expounded on the healing powers of nature as an antidote to the deleterious effects of industrialization and urban life. The Progressive Era, commonly defined as the period between 1890 and 1920, was marked by a number of social reform movements that aimed to improve sanitary conditions in urban areas, respond to the need for public green spaces, secure access to healthcare for citizens, and uplift the general moral standing of society through drug, alcohol, and sexual abstinence programs (Cooter and Pickstone 2020).

Reformers argued that industrialization had encumbered the overall well-being of populations, and a "return to nature" was an antidote to the social, moral, and bodily ills of the industrial era (Albanese 1986, 1993). By the 1860s, social reformers, or those who promoted specific changes to the sociopolitical structure of American society, claimed to have become disillusioned by the effects of industrialization on citizens' mental and physical health. Pollution from coal-burning factories filled the air, while raw sewage, factory runoff, animal carcasses, and improperly buried human remains leached into ground water, rivers, and other sources of drinking water. Environmentalist and conservation movements, each with different missions and goals, were generally concerned with abating the detrimental effects of industrialization on human health (Johnson 2018; Stradling 2004). Social reformers criticized the built environment, particularly cities, which they viewed as exceptionally dangerous, disease-ridden, and morally corrupt (Johnson 2018).

Progressive reformers and healers often invoked "nature" in ambiguous ways, as a polysemous category that "signified all things pure and simple in the natural world" (Albanese 1986: 490). "Nature" was also a metaphysical concept that referred to the experiential and causative power of the unseen; nature and God were congruent principles, and the healthy body was one that was in harmony with nature's laws (Albanese 1986: 491). For example, public hospitals for the insane often invoked a closeness to nature as a cure for a disorderly mind (Kuglitsch 2023: 188). Asylums, this perspective held, should be in natural settings and offer opportunities for outdoor recreating along paths, lawns, and gardens (Kuglitsch 2023). At the Western Washington Hospital for the Insane, patients participated in horticultural regimens meant to instill discipline and patience. Growing plants in greenhouses and then "planting them out" gave patients a predictable schedule, while rewards were offered for exceptional plant specimens. Patients also grew potted plants indoors, which, along with other domestic chores, habituated them to a calm life of domesticity. The different sizes of terra-cotta pots recovered from excavations at the hospital can be interpreted as *materia medica* insofar as they represent the significance of horticultural regimens for teaching patients discipline and self-control (Kuglitsch 2023). Both horticultural therapy and disciplinary schedules were meant to help patients recover from mental illness.

Other natural treatments (besides horticultural therapy) were popular with the masses during the nineteenth and early twentieth centuries. Different treatments included water (hydro) therapies or water cures, sun (helios) therapies, and air therapies (Whorton 2004), along with herbalism. Christian epistemologies of physiology also underpinned many natural medicinal systems, including hydropathy, Thomsonian medicine, and Transcendentalism (Johnston 2004). For many Christian sects, nature and God were congruent principles and the healthy body was that which was in harmony with nature's laws (Albanese 1986: 1). A quotation from *The Magnetic and Cold Water Guide* expounds the virtues of cold water therapy, stating that "instead of the dosing and drugging of the old system of practice, it proposes to rely on the indwelling healing power of nature alone, to provoke and regulate which, it employs the widespread element of fresh, unadulterated water" (Albanese 1986: 489).

Hydropathy, popularized during the early to mid-1800s, entailed a variety of healing methods such as drinking carbonated water, bathing in cold water at natural springs, or saunas (Legan 1971). Hydropathy was thought to cure a range of internal diseases and external afflictions, such as skin rashes and dermatitis (Cayleff 1991). Water cures were also advocated by physicians to treat gynecological issues (Cayleff 1991; Veit 1996). Physicians advocated sitz baths and vaginal douches during a woman's pregnancy and after delivery as a means of relieving pain (Veit 1996: 41). Archaeological research at the residences of Dr. Clifford Morrogh and Dr. Frank Donahue in New Jersey uncovered vaginal pessaries and syringes. These implements were likely used by the physicians to treat female patients using hydropathic medical treatments (Veit 1996: 41).

Although hydropathy was overwhelmingly limited to the middle and upper classes due to the necessity for leisure time to undertake such cures (Legan 1971), archaeological and documentary evidence indicates that working-class individuals did also participate in hydrotherapeutic practices. Linn's archaeological study of soda bottles from Five Points, New York, demonstrates the importance of water to the social identity and well-being of Irish immigrants. These Irish immigrants used soda water in ways reminiscent of practices in Ireland to remedy the physical, social, and economic ills that accompanied immigration to the United States (Linn 2010: 69). Soda bottles recovered from excavations at 472 and 474 Pearl Street in Five Points indicate the importance of soda water for treating a variety of physiological and spiritual afflictions. Medical reports from Bellevue Hospital in New York indicate that Irish-born patients outnumbered American- and German-born patients during the 1840s (Linn 2010: 74) and suffered from infectious diseases that included typhoid, cholera, malaria, and flu. Given the poor health outcomes of Irish immigrant residents of New York, it is not surprising that the residents of Pearl Street sought soda water remedies, which embodied both religious and secular modes of healing (Linn 2010: 89).

In addition to a "return to nature" (Whorton 2004), a general ethos of anti-intellectualism and populism pervaded nonprofessional sectors of medical practice throughout the 1800s and early 1900s (Flannery 2002). In particular, the Jacksonian era (1828–1854) was marked by a radical democratic philosophy: one grounded in the idea of the "common man" and the notion that one's intuitive wisdom and natural talents would ensure success (Flannery 2002: 443). As Flannery (2002) notes, "Jackson's election represented the fulfillment of a popular democratic spirit that emerged from complex socio-political and socioeconomic forces; western expansion, a wide-spread agrarian populace, and a broadly diffused fervent American Protestantism built upon a priesthood of all believers." While domestic and folk medicine date to the pre-Columbian and colonial periods in America, self-treatment was repopularized during the 1820s–1860s as "anti-authoritarian" approaches to medicine were fueled by anti-elitism and a general distrust of educated, middle- and upper-class professionals (Berman and Flannery 2001).

During the 1830s and 1840s, Jacksonian democratic ideals favored experience over education and ideology; as for medicine, "the nation faced a medical-education system that bordered on anarchy" (Haller 1981: 193). Jacksonian-period Americans were particularly open to nonorthodox medical treatments, such as homeopathy, Thomsonian medicine, hydropathy, and other forms of nonscientific medicine (Flannery 2002). In the 1830s and 1840s, most state legislatures, under pressure from anti-licensing proponents, removed any existing training and licensing restrictions on medical practice (Appel 2010). Samuel Thomson (1769–1843) was one of the most prolific and popular advocates of alternative medicine and self-care during the Jacksonian period (Fillmore 1986). Thomson had great disdain for professionally educated physicians, specifically for their supposed elitism and general lack of practical experience (Johnston 2004). Thomson argued that patients could self-treat if they had basic curative knowledge and access to botanical resources. He would travel to towns to consult with individual households and then sell the rights to practice Thomsonian medicine for twenty dollars (Johnston 2004). Rights in hand, an individual could join the Friendly Botanic Society, where members met to share experiences and medical information.

The popularity of Thomsonian medicine fueled the growth of "domestic medicine," especially among rural populations (Whorton 2004). Archaeological research conducted at the Hollywood Plantation in Arkansas demonstrates the importance of self-medication for farmers and their families (Barnes 2015). The plantation was owned and operated by a Dr. Taylor and his wife, Elizabeth Taylor, during the 1860s (Barnes 2015). Excavations near the back of the house and kitchen area revealed a large number of medicine bottles, most of which proclaimed themselves to be herbal treatments, including two glass bottle fragments of McElree's Wine of Cardui. Wine of Cardui was similar to Lydia Pinkham's Vegetable Compound, as it was used to treat "common female complaints" including fallen womb, inflammation, menstrual cramps, and general female pain. Elizabeth Taylor suffered miscarriages and stillbirths, dying in 1868 after her last child was born. The presence of Wine of Cardui bottles speaks to her desire to take control over her personal medical care and the healthcare of her family (Barnes 2015).

In sum, historical archaeological research has demonstrated the importance of alternative or nonheterodox preventative care methods and curative strategies for members of all sorts of American communities. Alternative medicines were integral to maintaining the health and well-being of marginalized communities, including Black Americans and other racialized and stigmatized groups. Household and community-based care practices, including herbalism and faith healing, performed dual roles, abating both the traumatic physical and psychosocial impacts of structural inequality and the marginalizing effects of an exclusionary professional healthcare sector. Other sectors of the American populace engaged in alternative medicine because they were distrustful of medical expertise, believed alternative medicine to be more effective than orthodox practices, or faced restricted access to professional care, whether economically or geographically. Alternative medicine, in all its varied instantiations, has commonly been relegated to the fringe by the professional medical sector. But as the archaeological and historical discussions in this chapter demonstrate, alternative medicine has been, and continues to be, a robust part of American lives.

Conclusion

Political reforms during the late nineteenth and early twentieth centuries had profound impacts on medical training, licensing, and the professionalization of medical practice, all of which significantly altered the American therapeutic landscape. Flexner's landmark report in 1910 resulted in the most sweeping medical training and education reforms in US history. The Flexner Report was precipitated by earlier developments in professional medicine. The late 1890s saw tremendous growth in state funding for biomedical research, new psychiatric hospitals, and healthcare support through company-sponsored insurance plans (Stahnisch and Verhoef 2012: 2). Scientific biomedical research was predominately funded by private corporations such as the Carnegie Foundation and Rockefeller Foundation (Berliner 1975). The closure of historically Black and homeopathic colleges after 1910, concerted efforts by the AMA to professionalize the field of medical practice, and private funding for biomedical research had profound and far-reaching impacts on the field of medicine. Paul Starr goes so far as to claim that by the 1920s in the United States, the authority of mainstream medicine was unchallenged and monolithic in scope (Starr 2017).

Medical historians have recently begun to question Starr's claim by critiquing the marginalized status of nonorthodox treatments among diverse American communities. As historian Johnston argues, scholars' task should be to historicize the complexities of alternative medical practices, rather than to write them off as anomalies in the face of standard medicine. In addition, "A complex rendering of American medical history in the twentieth century can shake off the ahistorical surprise that accompanies so many accounts of alternative medicine's 'comeback'" (Johnston 2004:

2). In the United States today, alternative practices to biomedicine exist, although the boundaries between CAM and biomedicine may not be sharp or fixed (Sikand and Laken 1998). As of 1993, one-third of Americans used at least one alternative therapy (Eisenberg et al. 1993); a comprehensive follow-up study in 2004 demonstrated that 62 percent of adults had used some form of CAM therapy over the course of twelve months (Barnes et al. 2004). CAM users have critiqued clinical medicine as reductive, mechanistic, and unsuccessful in treating chronic illness and mental health concerns (Eisenberg et al. 1998; Sikand and Laken 1998).

Historical archaeologists have made important contributions to the intellectual task of foregrounding the importance of so-called alternative therapies for racialized or ethnic minorities who are more likely to undergo discrimination and other negative experiences within the conventional medical system. Diverse communities have historically practiced nondominant modes of medicine as a response to exclusionary biomedical systems and to alleviate poor health outcomes. Alternative therapies were often based in long-standing cultural traditions and incorporated a set of diverse practices that drew from both ethnomedicine and scientific medicine (Johnson et al. 2019), as archaeologists have shown. Historical archaeologists have also called for new interpretive paradigms that avoid narrow ascriptions of health and healthcare behaviors. Seemingly nonmedical material culture, such as bathing paraphernalia, food preparation residues, and pins, index complex systems of care in which health-seeking behaviors permeated every aspect of one's life. Historical archaeological research highlights our own biases and limitations when seeking to understand contemporary healthcare practices. Archaeologists have called on researchers to expand their conceptual repertoire of medical objects and interpret them as significant players in people's social worlds. After all, as medical tools act as "vehicles of ideology, facilitators of self-care, and perceived sources of efficacy, they direct people's thoughts and actions and influence their social life" (van der Geest et al. 1996: 157).

3

Healthcare Consumerism and Medicalization

American consumers are inundated daily with pharmaceutical advertisements promising to address a range of health concerns, from high cholesterol to chronic depression, insomnia, erectile dysfunction, and beyond. While drug advertising in the United States is frequently directed at physicians and other healthcare providers, US drug companies increasingly spend on DTCA—which grew from $2.1 billion (11.9 percent) of total drug company spending in 1997 to $9.6 billion (32.0 percent) in 2016 (Schwartz and Woloshin 2019). DTCA has stirred debate among healthcare professionals, medical organizations, patients, advocacy groups, and governmental agencies (Donohue 2006; Donohue et al. 2007; Gellad and Lyles 2007). Opponents of DTCA disagree over the role of consumers in healthcare decision-making, the appropriateness of patient self-diagnosis, and the ethics of endorsing potentially harmful pharmaceuticals (Donohue 2006: 660). Practical and ethical questions regarding DTCA fundamentally concern the role of professional medical care in the lives of US patients and their transition from *patients* to *patient consumers* over the past century (Lyles 2002). Reasons for patients' health-seeking behaviors, including the shift to individual consumer models of healthcare, include unaffordable medical care costs and a general distrust in professional medical treatments (Lyles 2002). As medical professionals have argued, patients have increasingly moved away from the standard medical encounter, opting instead for self-care (Anderson et al. 2000).

The emergence of new medical marketplaces and patients' increasing identification as medical consumers have been described as contemporary occurrences (Anderson et al. 2000). But as the historical archaeological studies in this chapter demonstrate, self-care gained importance, as supported by material evidence that points to the commonality of self-care and alternative medicine for patients, as early as the eighteenth century and onward through the twentieth. Medical consumerism is not a late twentieth-century phenomenon; rather, the availability of patent or OTC drugs and drug advertising practices created a robust medical marketplace and a perceived need for certain drugs much earlier (Conrad and Leiter 2008).

This chapter integrates discussions about self-treatment and the significance of alternative medicine to highlight archaeological studies of patient consumerism. The sociopolitics of patient consumers—in other words, the idea that how people engage with medicine *shapes* and *is shaped by* their social and political worlds—are accessible to historical archaeological research. Archaeological studies have demonstrated how the presence of a robust medical marketplace during the nineteenth and early twentieth centuries facilitated patients' autonomy over their bodies and their care (Barnes 2015; Linn 2010; Wilkie 1996b). Cultural attitudes toward treatment and illness, democratic ideals concerning individual rights, and mass media and widespread advertising influenced how people engaged with healthcare marketplaces. Medical consumerism also anticipated the patient consumer rights activism of the 1960s and 1970s (Donohue 2006). Finally, archaeological research has shown that medicalization, or the creation of new pathologies and new health identities, is not a recent phenomenon but one that can be traced to patent medicine advertising and consumer practices in the nineteenth century. By addressing patterns of medicine consumption and consumerism, historical archaeologists have made important and timely contributions that show how the pharmaceutical industry shaped health ideals and influenced subjective understandings of health, illness, and the body.

Analyses of medicine consumerism and consumption in archaeology have played a crucial role in furthering our understanding of the relation between macro-scale processes, including medical advertising and political legislation, and micro-scale techniques of the body. Such studies have addressed three main phenomena: the role of pharmaceutical advertising in charting people's social and medical realities, how the patent medicine industry facilitated material practices associated with self-care, and how people resisted dominant ideologies of health via personal care practices. The historical relationships between consumerism and consumer agency, federal drug regulations, and drug advertising campaigns are important themes that have been addressed in historical archaeological studies of medicine. This chapter focuses on the sociopolitics of *patients as consumers* and the ways that historical archaeologists have addressed patterns of medicine consumption and medicine consumerism in their research. Topics in historical archaeological research include how professional organizations, legal regulations, healthcare agencies, and medical advertisements shape people's categorization of their physical bodies (normal or pathological), along with how medicine consumption shapes social identities (to include gender, sexuality, race, ethnicity).

Because of the fundamentally physical, individual, and often private act of medicine consumption, archaeologists are well positioned to push consumerism studies beyond frameworks of conspicuous consumption and to seriously consider how medicine consumption is integral to one's relationship with both the physical body and the social body (Scheper-Hughes and Lock 1987). Private medicine consumption differs from more overt, socially visible forms of consumption (Smith 2007), but it is greatly informed by advertising, medicalization discourses, and structural constraints. Thus, the act of consuming medicine relates to one's understanding of self, which is influenced by structural and ideological forces (Smith 2007).

This chapter begins by providing a brief review of consumption and consumerism studies in archaeology. Archaeological studies of medicine consumption and consumerism generally fall into three categories: (a) the affordances of the proprietary medicine industry in facilitating patients' self-care, (b) the role of pharmaceutical advertising in mapping people's social and medical realities through medicalization processes, and (c) patient resistance to dominant ideologies of health via self-care practices. Pharmaceutical advertising not only changed the way people consumed medication, but also played a fundamental role in medicalization processes, or the ways in which subjects thought about illness and health. Historical archaeological studies of medical advertisements and medicalization foreground the social and political contexts in which patients (or *patient consumers*) purchased medicines, used them, and conceived of their bodies and their health.

In the closing section of this chapter, I argue that archaeological studies of medicine consumption and consumerism are well positioned to contribute to contemporary critiques of patient-consumer models in healthcare policy and discourse. I draw on recent appraisals of medical consumerism by suggesting that "consumer choice" as an interpretive framework may overlook the complexity of medical practices, especially regarding self-care and self-medication. Patient choices about care are enacted in a dynamic world shaped by various and often competing forces. I argue that self-medication references continual processes of reconciling structural effects, materiality, and personal agency that archaeologists have addressed in their research.

Consumer Studies in Historical Archaeology

Studies of consumerism and consumption have figured large in the field of historical archaeology, both implicitly and explicitly. After all, archaeologists study what people *do* with the material world, including which items people make, buy, use, and then discard (Schiffer 1992). Archaeologists have drawn important distinctions between consumerism and consumption (Heath et al. 2017). Consumption refers to the individual act of using particular goods (Majewski and Schiffer 2009); this has been mobilized as an interpretive framework for explaining a range of actions evident in the archaeological record, from the relationship between supply and demand to the life course of an object, including its manufacture, use, and discard (Mullins 2011, 2012). Consumerism, on the other hand, refers to the socioeconomic contexts of consumption, which include product advertising and media, technology, webs of symbolism and meaning, and taste or fashion (Majewski and Schiffer 2009). Consumerism is an important medium through which individuals uphold their social identities and communicate their social, economic, and political positions via specific consumption activities (Orser 1994).

Historical archaeologists have demonstrated how eighteenth- and nineteenth-century consumers were not merely "duped" by capitalist ideologies, but incorporated commodities into their daily lives in ways that simulated specific forms of material agency (Harrison 2002; Wilkie 1996b) and distinguished themselves from other social groups (Shackel 1993). While recent trends in historical archaeology tend to foreground the social and performative aspects of consumerism, they build on earlier studies that seek to explain the relationships between consumer choice, social status, economic rank, and artifact patterning in the archaeological record (Spencer-Wood and Heberling 1987). As Heath and colleagues note (2017: 3), studying consumerism in historical archaeology requires archaeologists to consider the relationships between the material and ideological aspects of culture. If objects are symbolically meaningful for those who construct their social realities around them, and if they also have physical properties that limit and enable human action (Heath et al. 2017), then attending to this dependency is integral to understanding consumerism and consumption behavior.

Archaeological scholarship on consumer choice and commodity consumption generally falls under three related interpretive axes (Mullins 2011). Some scholars focus on the structural processes that restrain and enable particular consumption practices, such that consumers obtain and use specific goods in accordance with broader social, economic, and political influences. Other scholarship examines how individuals actively negotiate the meaning of things, and frequently develop consumption behaviors and symbolic meanings in direct opposition to dominant ideological and market forces (Mullins 2011). The third approach focuses on both structural forces and consumer agency by recognizing that "goods assume meaning in a tension between structural and localized processes that cannot be described as either wholly deterministic or disconnected from consumer symbolism" (Mullins 2011). These three interpretive frameworks will guide discussions of medicalization, healthcare consumerism, and resistance to medical models of consumption in the ensuing sections.

Self-Help and Self-Medication: Archaeologies of Medicine Consumption

The three axes identified by Mullins show how the social, economic, and political circumstances that created the conditions for "patient consumers" did not begin in the twentieth century, with managed care programs and patients' rights advocacy programs. Rather, the foundations of medical consumerism in the United States began with modern consumer capitalism, which changed the way patients sought doctors' care and medical drugs (Tomes 2016: 19). "Pay for service" models of medical care, drug advertising, and a wide variety of accessible pharmaceuticals available in the nineteenth century drastically altered patients' relationships to medical care.

The scarcity of formally trained physicians in the United States from the colonial period through the mid-1800s inspired a climate of self-help and domestic medicine. These approaches flourished as most patients sought assistance from physicians only as a last resort or for specialized surgical cases. Possibilities for self-medication and self-diagnosis expanded in the 1820s as literacy rates rose and technological advances in printing enabled households to purchase medical guides (Tomes 2016, 2021). Newspapers and medical guides became significant sources of medical information. In addition, new medical sects, such as homeopathic, Thomsonian, botanical, and homeopathic medicine, challenged the dominance and authority of university-trained doctors (Starr 2017). The prevalence of "do it yourself" medicine, alternative medical approaches, and a lack of state licensing laws and medical regulations occasioned a competitive and largely unregulated medical marketplace.

During the Progressive Era, 1890–1920, major social and political shifts in American politics transformed medical practice and self-treatment. First, patients' rights activists sought government regulations over the professional medical field (Starr 2017), which led to licensing and education requirements within professional medical practice. The second major shift centered around medical consumer protection laws. Progressive Era reformers addressed the potential dangers of medical commercialism, arguing that government oversight was necessary to protect consumers from potentially harmful drugs (Tomes 2016). Regulating the proprietary medicine market was difficult, since American companies had long thrived under a "free market" economy (Tomes 2016, 2020). Ironically, instead of creating a democratic relationship between patients and medical professionals, Progressive Era reforms of professional medicine during the late nineteenth century served to widen the gap between doctor and patient knowledge, drastically increase the cost of medical care, and inhibit access to professional medical care, particularly for rural, racially marginalized, and economically disadvantaged households (Tomes 2016: 91). Much to the chagrin of health reformers, the proprietary and patent medicine industry flourished by providing consumers with affordable and accessible healthcare alternatives (Bivins et al. 2016). Much like alternative medicines and OTC medications in the contemporary period, patent medicines provided an instrumental means of securing patient knowledge and bodily autonomy.

After the Civil War, drug manufacturers began to distinguish their products as either "ethical" or "patent" (Gabriel 2014). Ethical drugs had a known composition and were advertised to pharmacists and professional doctors (Starr 2017). *Patent medicine* is a colloquial term used to describe medical products produced by large companies during the nineteenth century that did not contain known or disclosed substances and were not targeted at the professional medical community. *Proprietary medicine* is a more general category of drugs that were not necessarily patented and contained secret preparations owned by individuals or companies (Street 1917; White 2021). Very few medicines on the nineteenth-century medical market were patented, and even fewer had been evaluated in processes similar to today's clinical trials (Young 2015).

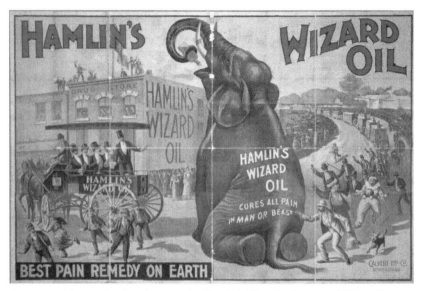

Figure 3.1. Lithograph advertisement for Hamlin's Wizard Oil, c. 1890. Wikimedia Commons, public domain.

The American patent medicine industry traces its roots to England in the early 1600s (Young 2015). Early patent medicine producers in England used print advertising to market their products (Young 2015: 4). The first medicine to be granted a patent in England was Anderson's Pills, whose manufacturer claimed to be a physician to King Charles I (Young 2015). American colonial populations continued to consume British patent medicines throughout the Revolutionary War period, but by the 1790s, apothecaries began refilling empty patent medicine bottles with their own remedies and American manufacturers started making their own products to undercut the cost of imported medicine (Young 2015: 15). During the eighteenth and nineteenth centuries, nearly every American household consumed some form of proprietary medicine. The patent and proprietary medicine industry was sustained through widespread marketing campaigns that included print materials and live-action sales shows (Figure 3.1) (White 2021: 516). By the 1850s, so-called patent medicines were a mainstay in most American households.

Patent medicine companies performed an imperative role in legitimizing patient health concerns, contributing to patients' medical knowledge, and affording patients a degree of autonomy over their care (Segal 2020). During the eighteenth and nineteenth centuries, many members of the public were distrustful of the invasive and often deadly treatments that most physicians offered. Self-help was an important alternative to receiving professional medical care (Conrad and Leiter 2008: 826). Patent medicine companies recognized the importance of these nonprofessional, pluralistic medical topographies and exploited them by developing mass-produced drugs that mimicked familiar home remedies (Conrad and Leiter 2008). While each patent medicine was marketed as a cure for a specific set of conditions, consumers often adapted them to suit their healthcare requirements, or in contemporary terms, for "off-label" use.

Historical archaeologists have shown how broader social, economic, political, and ideational forces have informed medicine consumption practices. This body of research also demonstrates how patient consumers recontextualized the meanings and intended uses of mass-produced medicines to meet their individual needs. These idiosyncratic and highly individualized choices precipitated new material practices. For example, archaeological research in the American South shows how African American consumers selected some mass-produced medical goods over others based on economic availability. Consumer choices were also driven by cultural beliefs concerning disease and treatment (Wilkie 1996b). African American women purchased readily available, affordable patent medicines "which best reflected their cultural ideals" (Wilkie 1996b: 120). Archaeological evidence of culturally grounded medicine consumption at Oakley Plantation, in Louisiana, includes medicine bottles and ointment jars. While mass-produced medicine bottles were more prevalent in later twentieth-century deposits, this does not necessarily indicate less dependence on African ethnomedical traditions. Looking closely at the composition of many of the commercially produced medicines from Oakley, they represent clear consumer preferences shaped by culture (Wilkie 1996b). For example, Vaseline, Moroline, and Bromo-Seltzer were used consistently by Oakley Plantation households (Wilkie 1996b: 125). The ingredients in these medications, such as peppermint and petroleum, stood in for traditional homeopathic remedies, such as the use of tallow to heal skin disorders or mint to cure stomach ailments. Vaseline and Moroline were also inexpensive and easily available products, significant for African American populations who were largely excluded from accessing professional care. Wilkie (1996b) argues that African Americans did not abandon ethnomedical traditions altogether in later periods but transformed them by selectively incorporating accessible proprietary medicines into preexisting cultural practices.

During the nineteenth century, urban inhabitants increasingly faced threats to their physical and mental welfare. Communities in industrialized areas were often exposed to communicable diseases, unsanitary conditions, and dangerous working conditions. Archaeological research conducted at the Courthouse Block in Five Points, New York, demonstrates how residents attempted to mitigate these threats. Unlike wealthier citizens of New York, who were geographically mobile and could afford preventative measures, such as residence at a sanatorium or attending public baths, occupants at Five Points relied on affordable home remedies and patent medicines (Bonasera and Raymer 2001). Artifact and macrobotanical analyses indicate that residents utilized ethical medicines (those prescribed by a physician), patent medicines, herbal remedies, and soda water to mitigate the ill effects of urban life (Bonasera and Raymer 2001). Due to economic constraints, most households would have obtained ethical medicines from a variety of sources, including dispensaries, hospitals, and apothecary shops.

Archaeologists have also examined how ethnicity, religion, and community belonging helped shape culturally bounded notions of health, thus influencing consumer behavior. Linn's research into healthcare has shown how cultural traditions shape health-seeking behaviors. In New York, Irish immigrant families suffered from higher rates of contagious and noncontagious illnesses than German- and American-born families (Linn 2010: 74). During the 1800s, water healing, or "hydropathy," was an important form of homeopathic treatment that purported to cure chronic and infectious diseases such as respiratory infections and stomach disorders (Linn 2010). Bathing, drinking natural sparkling or flavored water, and steam treatments were among the more popular water cures. Soda water from natural springs was advertised as a cure for both infectious diseases and chronic conditions. Irish immigrants adopted soda water in culturally familiar ways in order to ameliorate physical, social, and economic hardship in America (Linn 2010: 84). Linn (2010) argues that soda water likely "stood in" for Irish holy wells and spring waters as spiritual, bodily, and psychological cures.

At Five Points, mineral water bottles were common in the artifact assemblage, indicating that soda water consumption was particularly meaningful to newly arrived Irish immigrants; they would have been familiar with the religious and healing powers of water (Bonasera and Raymer 2001; Linn 2010). In America, advertisements claimed that mineral and soda waters could cure symptoms associated with digestive failures, bronchitis, asthma, skin diseases, diabetes, mental strain, and physical excesses (Yamin et al. 1997: 50). Soda water, an inexpensive remedy, would have "satisfied the local proponents of temperance, who saw mineral water as an appropriate substitute for alcohol" (Yamin et al. 1997: 50). Consumer medicine choices at Five Points reflected a number of related variables, from culturally significant practices associated with water to economic status and purchasing power, along with one's lived experiences and familiarity with certain types of treatments.

Historical archaeological research on Chinese railroad workers' healthcare practices in the American West similarly shows cosmopolitan practices involving both Chinese and Euro-American medicines. Chinese medical theories of the body include a complex array of ontologies regarding the elements and qualities necessary for maintaining health (Heffner 2015). Imbalances between elements within and outside the body led to disease, which necessitated the application of internal and external remedies. Heffner (2015) notes that plants, foods, and minerals could be used in both external and internal treatments to treat diseases. In North America during the nineteenth century, Chinese doctors in urban environments treated both Chinese American and Euro-American patients for stomach complaints, tumors, blood disorders, consumption, and asthma (Heffner 2015: 136). Documentary sources on Chinese medicine in the United States reflect a formal system of medicine practiced by doctors who gained medical training through apprenticeship or university education. However, workers in railroad and mining camps would not have had access to Chinese doctors and urban medicine stores. Instead, archaeological evidence from railroad sites dating to 1865–1910 indicates that Chinese workers engaged in informal consumer strategies and medical pluralism (Heffner 2015). Patent medicines found at these sites include bitters, tonics, liniments, sarsaparillas, and extracts. Other artifacts include Chinese medicine vials, opium-smoking paraphernalia, kegs for storing tea, and implements used to perform skin scraping and skin modification (Heffner 2013, 2015). Chinese railroad workers made healthcare choices that reflected a basic knowledge of Chinese medical theory and practice as well as European and American patent medicines. Healthcare practices in remote locations among Chinese immigrant communities were diversified and strategic, incorporating elements of practice that were culturally familiar and easily accessible.

As the archaeological case studies in this section demonstrate, patent medications were used by patients as a strategy to take control over their healthcare and to overcome perceived medical gatekeeping (Talevi 2010). Today, patients' access to pharmaceuticals is increasingly framed as a form of patient autonomy, a growing rejection of medical paternalism, and the democratization of access to medical information and medical products (Donohue 2006). While access to medical information and healthcare resources are touchpoints for debates concerning patients' rights in the contemporary moment, eighteenth- and nineteenth-century patients' rights discourses similarly touted the importance of private enterprise, self-care, and patient knowledge (Tomes 2016). Some of the earliest medical manuals available in America foregrounded the importance of medical knowledge, self-care, and a spirit of autonomy (Zebroski 2016). Self-empowerment discourses and practices were buttressed by the wide variety and availability of patent medicines and home cures during the nineteenth century (Segal 2020). Archaeological research demonstrates how a robust patent medicine market helped patients overcome negative health outcomes, deal with poverty and discrimination, and seek out alternatives to an increasingly exclusionary professional medical field. As the archaeological studies in this section show, home healthcare and patent medicines were invaluable resources for marginalized and minoritized patients. Furthermore, a close attention to context shows that patent medicines and natural remedies, such as soda waters, were adapted by patients to accommodate their culturally grounded healthcare needs. This pushes archaeologists to critically evaluate the context and use life of objects that do not immediately appear "medical," but were nonetheless significant to people's self-care regimes.

Patient Consumerism in Historical Archaeology

Federal Drug Regulation

It is important to note that the patent medicine industry did not remain unencumbered by federal regulation. Weighing the medical market against the market for other consumer products, medical professionals and patients' rights advocates saw the former as potentially more dangerous than the latter (Musto 1999; Tomes 2016). The pharmaceutical market represents a complex nexus of power between federal and state government agencies, drug companies and the pharmaceutical industry, and patients. Importantly, patients' rights to medical knowledge and resources, as well as patient competency, were significant stimuli for policies concerning drug regulation.

Despite the popularity of patent medicines and their widespread use during the nineteenth and twentieth centuries, they were not exempt from critique by professional medical organizations. The AMA criticized the patent medicine industry for being irresponsible with patient consumers (Boyle 2013). The AMA recognized that the sale and advertising of medicines were distinctly different from other kinds of products, given that medicines directly impacted public health (Cramp 1911). Doctors critiqued the sale of patent medicines on the grounds that patients were not adept at measuring the effects and consequences of taking them. Doctors stated that patients were incapable of determining whether they had gotten better as a result of taking a medicine or in spite of it (Cramp 1911); they also argued that patients were particularly susceptible to false and misleading advertising. Advertising discourses often aimed to convince otherwise healthy individuals that they needed to self-medicate, thus increasing medicine sales. As Arthur Cramp (1911: 757), director of the Propaganda for Reform Department of the AMA, stated, "No man has any moral right to so advertise as to make well persons think they are sick and sick persons think they are very sick. Such advertising is an offence against the public health."

In 1906, the US Congress enacted the Pure Food and Drug Act, which hastened the creation of the Food and Drug Administration (FDA) (Musto 1999). The act required that manufacturers include dangerous or addictive product ingredients on product packaging (Donohue 2006). In accordance with the act, drug advertisers could not make intentionally false claims, nor could they specifically list the diseases a drug was intended to treat (Donohue 2006; Starr 2017). The act also recognized the *United States Pharmacopeia,* a manual produced by university-trained physicians and pharmacists, as the standard for drugs (White 2021: 516). Prior to 1938, physicians had the authority to write prescriptions for proprietary medicines, but a prescription was not needed in order for patients to acquire drugs from a pharmacy (Temin 1980). It is also important to note that while patent and proprietary medicines were often developed by university-trained physicians and pharmacists, they were not required to undergo scientific evaluations (White 2021: 519).

Archaeological research demonstrates how changing federal regulations, along with professional perceptions of patent and proprietary medicines, altered the relationship between patients and the medical marketplace. By the twentieth century, advocacy work on the part of physicians, journalists, and government agencies led to government oversight and control over the advertising and distribution of patent medicines (White 2021: 519). By the beginning of the twentieth century, medical training requirements, clinical trials, applied research, and highly publicized patent medicine deaths and addictions convinced many members of the American public that trained doctors and pharmacists provided safer and effective services (White 2021: 520).

Historical archaeological research, such as that at the Alameda-Stone Cemetery Site in Tucson, Arizona, has demonstrated the effects of medicine regulation for practitioners and medical consumers. Medicine-related artifacts at this site provide important information on the types of ailments that residents treated and suggest that residents purchased patent and professionally compounded medicines to treat their illnesses (White 2021: 532). Professional doctors were few in Tucson until the 1860s. The professionalization of the Tucson medical community accelerated in 1873, when the Arizona Legislature passed a law that would fine any unqualified person that practiced medicine. The formation of the Arizona Medical Association in 1892 further legitimized university-trained doctors and pharmacists in the territory.

Archaeological excavations at the Alameda-Stone Cemetery Site recovered 1,405 medicine-related artifacts and patent medicine bottles, which represented nationally popular products. A small number of prescription bottles in the assemblage provide information on the Tucson pharmacists that filled medical prescriptions for residents. Two of the prescription bottles retained their contents, which provided the opportunity to study professionally compounded historical period medicines. The recovery of medicine bottles with their original contents intact is common in historical archaeology, and chemical analyses of proprietary and patent medicines have demonstrated their specific makeup and their potential efficacy (Torbenson et al. 2000; von Wandruszka and Warner 2018; Voss et al. 2015). Furthermore, medicine bottles can provide useful information on medicine use in light of changing sociopolitical circumstances and the development of scientific medical knowledge. White (2021) and collaborators subjected these bottles' contents (liquid and hand-rolled pills) to mass spectrometry analysis. Compounds detected in the liquid medicine included camphor, phenol, and palmitic acid, all components that were effective and widely used in compounded medicines during the nineteenth century. Data from the Alameda-Stone Cemetery Site indicates that while medical professionals in the Arizona territory worked to decrease the proliferation of patent medicines, Tucson residents continued to use them. Furthermore, the presence of professionally compounded medicine indicates that pharmacists in Tucson used effective ingredients and "time tested cures" (White 2021: 538). This study, in addition to other earlier archaeological examples (Brighton 2005; Howson 1993; Linn 2010), demonstrates many communities' continuing preference for patent medicines.

Advertising, Medicalization, and the Patent Medicine Industry

Medical advertising and the wide availability of medicines shaped healthcare practices and people's material realities, but they also influenced the ways that patients thought about their own health. Medical advertising, particularly DTCA, helped to simultaneously create an emerging disease landscape and a burgeoning array of medical consumers who were driven to treat new and emerging diseases. By advertising directly to patients, patent medicine companies aimed to increase profits through a) informing patients about diseases and treatments they might have been unaware of, or even did not know they suffered from; b) aggressively encouraging patients to interface with medical providers about potential treatments; and c) introducing a wider range of so-called lifestyle drugs. Patent medicine advertising campaigns were a contentious, yet highly effective, means by which patients acquired healthcare knowledge and advice and turned this knowledge into consumer power. While DTCA is typically regarded as a twentieth-century phenomenon, pharmaceutical advertising has a much longer history in the United States (Lyles 2002). During the nineteenth and early twentieth centuries, patent medicine consumer practices mirrored the coterminous growth of drug advertising and medical markets that ensured their sales and success (Conrad and Leiter 2008). The development of new medical technologies, treatments, and drugs sparked interest among the general population, while advertising increased consumer demand and shaped how medical consumers thought about health and their own bodies.

Medicine consumption is a social process influenced by experience, knowledge, and the interpretation of information from various sources, including drug advertisements (Kamat and Nichter 1998; Vuckovic and Nichter 1997). "Medicalization" is the process whereby previously nonmedical problems are defined as medical ones, usually in terms of disease or disorders (Conrad and Leiter 2008: 825). The agents of medicalization include the medical profession, the market (drug companies, advertisers, and consumers), and patient advocacy groups. The development and promotion of new medical technologies, the emergence of new medical markets, and consumer demand driven by patient knowledge and patient choice have all shaped medicalization (Vuckovic and Nichter 1997). Exploring the tensions between structural forces (such as availability, pricing, and marketing and advertising) and consumer agency (individual and cultural values, how people socialize material goods, and symbolic use) represents a productive conceptual framework from which to examine advertising and the material effects of consumer behavior (Mullins 2012: 3). The following sections explore the concept of medicalization by offering historical and archaeological case studies to demonstrate how drug companies mobilized visions of health and illness that created new medical markets and consumer practices.

DTCA played an essential role in medicalization by pathologizing previously nonmedical conditions and simultaneously creating the need for a product to treat these conditions. Through medical advertising, patent medicine companies created perceived needs for products that assuaged consumers' fears about their bodies (Conrad and Leiter 2008). Patent medicine companies developed advertisements that claimed to treat a panoply of common afflictions by using new medical terms and language while at the same time distancing themselves from the professional medical community. Research on medicalization in anthropology demonstrates the usefulness of tracing the ways in which cultural values, collective anxieties, and marketing practices shape the consumption of medicine (Moynihan 2002; Nichter 1996). In the case of patent medicine advertising, health concerns were elaborated by pharmaceutical marketing strategies that played upon collective fears and indexed specific cultural values (Conrad and Leiter 2008). Pharmaceutical advertisements claimed to alleviate the stresses of industrial life, since the effects of urbanization, change in labor routines, and time demands became of increasing concern to patients during the nineteenth century. Advertisements shaped how medical consumers thought about their bodies, the presence of disease and experience of illness, and their own health identities (Ryzewski 2007).

Medicalization involves top-down processes by which *physical* conditions come to be defined and treated specifically as *medical* conditions (Conrad 1992; Moynihan 2002), which makes them objects of study, diagnosis, intervention, and treatment. Scholars have identified medicalization as a critical framework for exploring the relationships between consumer advertising, pharmaceutical development, and individuals' self-identification *as patients* with specific conditions (Nye 2003). During the nineteenth century, patent medicine manufacturers developed targeted advertisements that encouraged patients to self-diagnose and self-medicate with at-home cures. In their advertisements, patent medicines encouraged consumers to medicalize everyday problems, such as tiredness, nervousness, pain, and indigestion (Conrad and Leiter 2008: 826). Patent medicine manufacturers recognized that they could create a demand for certain products by first instilling the fear of disease or sickness in potential consumers (Young 2015: 184). Their medicines came to represent the literal cures for fast-paced, modern life: "Medicine manufacturers didn't collect orders and then fill them, as was the practice with other goods. Rather, they created a steady supply of the product, and then generated the demand" (Anderson 2004: 11). For example, a nineteenth-century advertisement for Burdock Blood Bitters claimed that "there are thousands of females in America who suffer untold miseries from chronic diseases common to their sex" (Segal 2020). This gendered language appealed to women consumers who perceived themselves as belonging to a broader community of patients who were often excluded from professional care, or whose bodies and ailments were stigmatized in professional medical encounters.

Gender, Medicine Consumption, and Medicalization

Women's health conditions were often misconstrued or stigmatized by physicians, as doctors overwhelmingly perceived women as "prisoners of their reproductive systems" (Bashford 1998). Because of this, women were often reticent to seek (male) physicians' assistance. Proprietary and patent medicines offered women a refuge from male doctors and professional therapies, since patent medicine companies claimed to offer women an opportunity to take responsibility for their own health (Larsen 1994). In fact, patent medicine advertisements' messaging regarding women's health was ambivalent. On one hand, advertisements expounded the importance of women's agency over their own health concerns. On the other, patent medicine advertisements mirrored nineteenth-century medical arguments that reified stereotypes about women, such as passivity, domesticity, and morality, and claimed that these traits were biologically grounded in women's physiology (Marcellus 2008). By drawing from cultural tropes that referenced the Victorian era's "cult of domesticity," nineteenth-century medical advertisements reinforced dominant ideologies that positioned women as the primary caretakers of the home (Larsen 1994). Advertisements for medicines reinforced gendered labor norms by claiming to treat

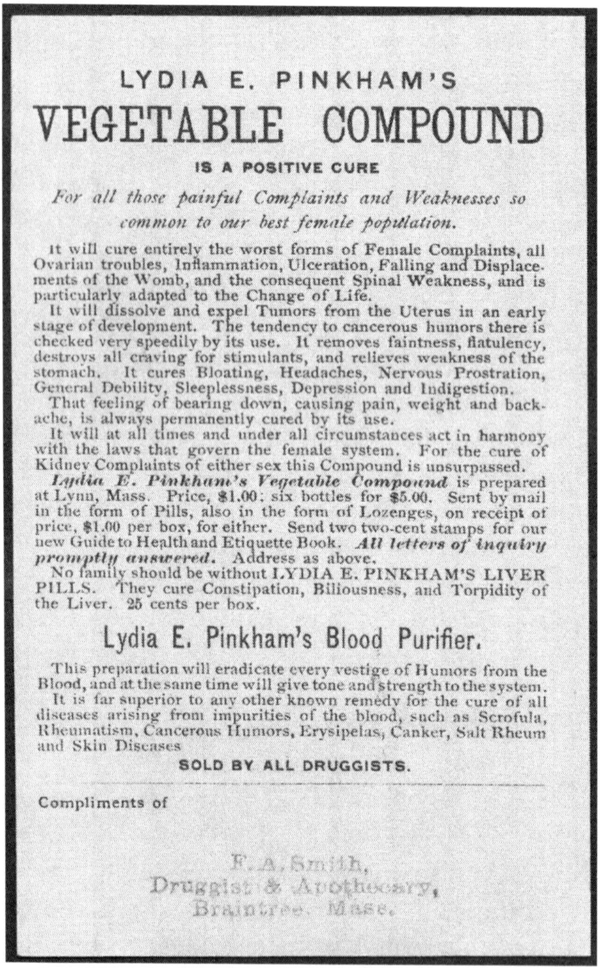

Figure 3.2. Lydia Pinkham's Vegetable Compound trade card, 1870–1900. Wikimedia Commons, public domain.

conditions and ailments that were considered specific to women's bodies and their roles as wives, mothers, and caretakers (Figure 3.2).

During the Progressive Era (1890–1920), patent medicine advertising language mirrored changing gendered societal expectations. Ads for patent medicines increasingly targeted the "working woman" by developing products that could treat the symptoms of factory work and other forms of labor that took place outside the home. For example, Lydia Pinkham's Vegetable Compound claimed to "strengthen the back and pelvic organs, bringing relief and comfort to tired women who stand all day in the home, shop, or factory" (Conrad and Leiter 2008: 828). By the 1920s, popular magazines for women such as *Good Housekeeping* and *Ladies' Home Journal* ran health-related articles that dispensed information on topics from childcare to beauty and feminine hygiene, while avoiding more galvanizing and ostensibly immoral topics such as gynecology and birth control (Conrad and Leiter 2008: 546; Segal 2020). Ironically, the lack of substantive women's health information in journal articles meant that women often turned to advertisements in the very same journals for medical advice. These advertisements were part of aggressive marketing campaigns that focused on pain relievers and feminine hygiene products (Segal 2020). Medicine companies used scientific-sounding language to market themselves as leading lights in the medical science field, while advertisements for specific products purported to address a range of domestic and personal needs. For example, the manufacturers of Lysol stated that the product could sanitize one's nursery, kitchen, and toilet and act as a vaginal antiseptic all at the same time (Conrad and Leiter 2008: 464).

Archaeological research has demonstrated how women responded to the information promoted by marketing campaigns and negotiated the medicalization of their own health. Barnes's (2015) archaeological study of nineteenth-century household medicine at the Hollywood Plantation in rural Arkansas explores the intersections between gender, advertising and medicalization, and self-medication. Barnes mobilizes Foucault's theories of biopower to understand how women in the Taylor family at the Hollywood Plantation responded to DTCA and the medicalization of everyday health conditions. Medicine company advertising influenced how members of the Taylor family perceived their bodies and health statuses (Barnes 2015). But family members also became agentive actors in this same medicalization process by performing certain self-treatment and personal care strategies. Eight of the patent medicines found at Hollywood were marketed to women and promoted as treating illnesses "particular to their sex" (Barnes 2015), such as Wine of Cardui, which was advertised as a treatment for women's ailments like menstrual pain and tiredness. Medicines found at Hollywood helped women in the family negotiate complex and changing gender roles, manage physical pain and anxieties concerning their health, and treat gynecological conditions that they could not openly discuss with professional doctors. Other items from Hollywood, such as cosmetic products, perpetuated gendered, racialized, and classist beauty ideals. Cosmetic advertisers upheld the idea that youth, natural beauty, and pale skin were the standards of beauty for middle- and upper-class women (Downing 2012). Given the presence of cosmetics at Hollywood, women of the household appear to have made choices to maintain their reproductive health and physical beauty by utilizing products that specifically targeted reproduction and aging as something to be avoided, or at least managed (Barnes 2015).

Other historical archaeological research shows how women interpreted cultural ideas about their bodies and refuted dominant ideologies through their engagement with certain medications and medical devices. Medicine bottles and childcare devices recovered from nineteenth-century privies at Harpers Ferry National Historical Park, West Virginia, suggest that mothers at the site negotiated gendered cultural ideals regarding motherhood (Larsen 1994). Instead of reaffirming reductionist and medicalizing theories regarding women's natural, biological status as mothers, certain care objects may have freed women from these dominant ideologies. Care and medicine objects from Harpers Ferry include a nursing bottle, whooping cough remedy, and Pitcher's Castoria bottles (a castor oil alternative). Larsen (1994) argues that hand-feeding infants with nursing bottles freed women from the constraints of breastfeeding. Cures for childhood diseases, such as whooping cough medicine and Castoria, could have been purchased from local pharmacies instead of relying on professional care from doctors (Larsen 1994: 76). By using these care products, women took command of their roles as mothers and caregivers in ways that offered them flexibility and control. In closing, Larsen argues that the challenge for historical archaeologists who study gendered practices, gendered ideals, and medicine is to attend to how women in the past negotiated gender roles. Medicines for children's diseases and feeding bottles may superficially indicate the presence of women at a site or may indicate that women adopted idealized nineteenth-century gender roles. But by paying close attention to context and how these items were used, archaeologists may interpret how motherhood practices actually "extended" gender roles and how proprietary medicines and medical technologies offered alternative treatment and care options for women (Larsen 1994).

Hygiene products for women similarly signaled gendered social and political fears about illness. One oft-cited example of how women's bodies become medicalized is through menstrual products and advertising (Liu et al. 2021). Advertising for menstrual products can be dated to the early 1800s (Smith 2007). By the late 1800s, disposable products for menstruation took on new symbolic meanings in keeping with Progressive Era social values of women as "clean" and as keepers of family health (Park 1996). "Sanitary products" (as they are still known today) heralded values of both cleanliness and secrecy in regard to women's bodies. Disposable sanitary towels and sanitary clothes were white, so that soiled examples could easily be "dealt with" through disposal or washing (Smith 2007: 424). The medicalization of women's reproductive cycles through advertising both created a need for certain products and pathologized menstruation as something "dirty" and in need of fixing.

The historical discussions and archaeological case studies presented in this section demonstrate how medicine advertising, medicalization, and medicine consumption are relational and active processes. By "disease mongering," or creating a recognized need for drugs to treat previously unknown diseases, companies created new social realities of the body and shaped the nineteenth-century disease landscape. Advertising created standards for health, well-being, and hygiene, and these expectations were experienced by individuals who accepted, negotiated, or rejected wholesale these normative health standards (Ryzewski 2007: 21). Medicine advertising and popular discourses were an important source of medicalization, or the transformation of "normal" bodily conditions into pathological ones. As archaeological research has shown, medicalization discourses provided information to consumers and shaped purchasing practices, ultimately influencing how they treated their own bodies. Archaeological studies also historicize drug companies' long-standing relationship with consumer behavior and consumers' health identities. Today, prescription medications, OTC drugs, and dietary supplements claim to provide patients control over their healthcare and serve to materialize health identities. For example, someone who takes medicine for a chronic condition or specific disease is a "patient" who identifies with that particular condition. By consuming certain medications, patients affirm a particular course of action and a specific subject position. This process requires that patients recognize themselves as "medicated selves" with particular conditions that are necessarily tied to their physical identities (Smith 2007: 419).

It is also important to note that medicalization is not a uniform, top-down process; consumers may resist medicalized visions of their physiological selves or adapt certain medicines in ways that make sense to them. Reasons for abstaining from drug use include not wanting to be socially or self-identified as "infirm," wanting to avoid drug dependency, and not wanting to take too many medications (Smith 2007: 419). Other individuals may resist social norms by altering treatment methods or refusing them altogether, thus avoiding self-ascription as a patient with a specific medical condition (Conrad 1992). Finally, as archaeological case studies in this section demonstrate, the sociopolitics of medicine consumption is not a recent phenomenon; it is entrenched in historical standards of health and wellness along with advertising campaigns and strategies, all of which have long been negotiated by individuals in their everyday lives.

Medicine Consumption as Resistance to Dominant Health Ideals

Medical anthropologists have contributed significant insights into techniques by which bodies have been colonized, medicalized, and commodified through medical practices (Panter-Brick and Eggerman 2018). Archaeologists have also made important contributions to this conversation about power and medicine by showing how material practices operate through technologies of normalization that facilitate the classification and control of bodies. Given the contingent nature of power, individuals and communities can resist normalizing strategies and refute dominant models of what it means to be "healthy." Health ideals and practices often extend beyond the dominant biophysical models suggested by government organizations and corporate standards (Adelson 2000). There are often disparities between biomedical standards of health and personal understandings of well-being, pointing to a multitude of variegated practices and values associated with how one views one's health within diverse historical, social, political, spiritual, and environmental states. Health is not a universal fact or state of being but "a constituted social reality" (Saltonstall 1993: 12). For example, communities may define "health" according to a complex nexus of mental well-being, spiritual health, and physical wellness (Adelson 2000).

This section focuses on how individuals have actively negotiated prevailing definitions of *health* by adopting consumer behaviors in opposition to dominant ideological forces. Social and political institutions often narrowly define *health* as physical fitness or aptitude (McGillivray 2005). Conversely, subjective definitions of what it means to be healthy may be guided by physical, psychological, or spiritual concerns, and are thus contextually dependent. Furthermore, individual health consumerism often reflects different values and ideologies than those promoted by people in positions of power. For example, archaeological research conducted at the Lowell Boardinghouse in Massachusetts reveals how various subjective definitions of health and well-being influenced healthcare decisions by Boott Mills workers. At Lowell Boardinghouse, workers rejected dominant corporate definitions of health and associated healthcare practices (Mrozowski et al. 1989). During the nineteenth century, concepts of health and well-being tended to be class-based and grounded in moral concerns (Beaudry 1993;

Mrozowski et al. 1989). By the nineteenth century, the deleterious effects of urbanization, pollution, and factory labor were thoroughly politicized. Middle- and upper-class reformers viewed sickness as a moral failing insofar as disease targeted those who practiced unhygienic behaviors, who failed to prevent disease, and who did not practice commonly accepted standards of healthy behavior (Mrozowski et al. 1989).

As Beaudry (1993) argues, working-class people commonly developed ideals of well-being that directly contradicted middle- and upper-class understandings of health. Workers tended to define well-being as the freedom to participate in restful leisure activities that did not necessarily meet corporate definitions of physiological health or physical fitness (Beaudry 1993: 92). At Boott Mills, corporate concern for worker fitness (and thus, productivity) was grounded in middle-class values concerning alcohol and tobacco abstinence and "healthy" eating. But these dominant ideals contrast starkly with archaeological evidence from worker housing areas. Zooarchaeological analyses suggest that according to modern standards, workers consumed relatively "boring" and nonnutritious foods: large quantities of fatty meats and carbohydrates (Beaudry 1993; Mrozowski et al. 1989). Documentary evidence shows that workers deemed their meals nutritious and adequately appetizing, prioritizing filling meals full of carbohydrates and fats. While factory labor and poor living conditions at Boott Mills had an undeniable effect on workers' physiological health, capitalist promises to "buy back health" by consuming medicines, abstaining from alcohol and tobacco, and following a restricted diet did not noticeably shape workers' healthcare choices. Instead, workers performed subjective understandings of health by consuming different kinds of "comfort" foods and social drugs such as tobacco and alcohol (Mrozowski et al. 1989). Well-being means different things to different people; the material manifestations of these meanings, evident in the archaeological record, can be used to interpret these different value systems (Beaudry 1993: 93).

Lee's (2017) investigation of health consumerism at the Poplar Forest plantation in Virginia highlights how issues of racialization, medicalization, and exploitation shaped enslaved people's experiences of care and well-being. Lee (2017: 141) uses the concept of "health consumerism" to refer to patients' involvement in their own care and the degree of economic freedom African Americans had to shape their health experiences. Enslaved healers made healthcare choices within the restraints of plantation slavery and a dominant white healthcare system. They modified African practices to incorporate European and Native American influences and adapt to new social, economic, and physical situations (Lee 2017: 143). Lee's analysis focuses on historical and archaeological data from the mid-1800s and evidences changing cultural ideas concerning disease etiologies and methods of treatment. Macrobotanical remains recovered from an enslaved cabin at Poplar Forest provide evidence concerning the diet and medicinal practices of enslaved households. A range of local, nonlocal, wild, and domesticated plant taxa suggest that enslaved people relied on their ethnobotanical knowledge for nutrition and healing purposes (Lee 2017: 145). Enslaved healers also incorporated aspects of spiritual care, as evidenced by the presence of crystals and other minerals used in conjuring practices. Patent medicine bottles, proprietary medicine bottles, and soda water bottles were also recovered from the cabin, indicating that enslaved people utilized diversified healthcare strategies. In sum, enslaved people's medicinal practices were grounded in a general belief that the whole body must be treated (physical body, spirit, community), which contrasted to planters' definition of the health of the enslaved as constituting physical fitness and aptitude for work.

As Ryzewski (2007: 17) notes, medicines and healthcare products are infused with multiple meanings and situated within individual cultural negotiations. Archaeological studies of health consumerism and medicine consumption have explored the tensions between consumer choice, advertising, medicalization, and symbolic meaning. By focusing on the complex and historically contextual relationships between advertising, medicalization, and medicine consumption, archaeologists have contributed to a broader understanding of how the pharmaceutical industry shaped individual ideals and perceptions of health, illness, and the body.

Archaeological research has shown how medical markets developed as early as the eighteenth century, as patent medicines became popular among marginalized communities and/or those who chose not to engage with the professional medical field. Despite these medicines' popularity, the companies that produced them perpetuated certain classist, gendered, and racist tropes that pathologized the bodies of working-class people, women, and racialized minorities. Patent medicine companies medicalized everyday conditions, such as tiredness or women's reproductive issues, to create a broad base of "patient consumers." Individuals were active participants in these newly created "medical markets," but they could also eschew these practices and definitions altogether. At the Hollywood Plantation, medicalization discourses shaped women's consumer behavior: they used products that were specifically designed to treat "women's ailments" along with cosmetics that purported to keep women looking young and vigorous. In Tucson, Arizona, nineteenth-century residents consistently purchased proprietary medicines to treat common diseases despite the prevalence of available pharmacies and doctors. Proprietary medicines and advertising thus shaped consumer decisions and subjective understandings of treatment and health, as well as affording patients autonomy over their own care. Finally, medical consumerism is a contested and power-laden field of practice. Decisions concerning how and how often to care for bodies depend on prevailing notions of health and sickness. As demonstrated by the final archaeological studies in this chapter, patient consumers often eschewed dominant ideologies of health and participated in healthcare practices that best fit their own subjective understandings of health and well-being.

Conclusion: Are Medical Patients Really Consumers?

As Tomes (2006: 83) argues, "Managed care organizations call people *consumers* so they don't have to think of them as *patients*." Deliberately booking a doctor visit, visiting a pharmacy, and participating in prescribed methods of care are all expected modes of practice within the world of modern medicine. The current configuration of the US healthcare system requires that patients make skillful choices that save personal costs, get good care, and ultimately keep themselves healthy (Tomes 2006). In the United States, patients with chronic conditions are expected to self-regulate, engage in self-care, and take responsibility for their own well-being (Tomes 2007). Since the 1990s, managed care programs have sought to cut medical care spending by limiting consumers' "shopping options." Scholars have argued that patients who choose out-of-network doctors and hospitals and who pay out of pocket for medications are engaged in a process through which they must choose highly beneficial yet less costly options (Tomes 2006). The contemporary patient-as-consumer model, born of individualism and economic incentives, envisions patients as the gatekeepers of their own health. Managed care programs state that they promote patient autonomy and medical expertise, transferring the balance of power from physicians to patients. But shopping for medical services is not the same thing as shopping for other material commodities, such as cars and trinkets. And those who are sick and/or deem themselves in need of medical care rarely initiate consumer behavior and experience medical markets in the same way as nonmedical consumers.

The contemporary professional sector of the American healthcare system is organized around three modes of access that combine private insurance, clinics and hospitals, and at-home care. Unlike other Western nations, which provide compulsory health insurance or have instituted comprehensive national health services, America has relied on private enterprise, from private insurance companies to corporate hospitals, private pharmaceutical companies, and until recently, physicians who were able to charge what they wished for their services (Tomes 2016). The US healthcare system has also fostered an unusual situation in which patients have come to be conceptualized quite narrowly as "patient consumers." This definition relates to a wide swath of the American public and generally refers to individuals who are responsible for ensuring their own care and health status. The historical celebration of economic liberty over social welfare concerns has shaped a unique healthcare system in which the rhetoric of "consumer choice" is frequently mobilized in medical practice (Tomes 2006).

Critics of the medical patient-consumer model have argued that it is unsuitable for actually providing healthcare, since the ideal of the informed, self-aware, and liberal subject who can choose from a range of options is deeply flawed in this context. The concept of "medical markets" in the United States has been described as an anomaly since medical markets (if they can be so called) do not meet the standards of competitive marketplaces (Tomes 2006). Contemporary patient consumers are limited by federal legislation, health insurance policies, and time and economic constraints. Medicine development and marketing, along with physician licensing and education requirements, have been adjudicated by the federal government since the late nineteenth century. Other critics of patient-consumer models have argued that transferring the onus of care onto patients absolves healthcare professionals and organizations of responsibility and unduly burdens already sick patients (Goldstein and Bowers 2015). Patient-led care often does not grant patients autonomy, nor does it respect individual decision-making regarding healthcare. Rather, patient-consumer models elide the structural constraints that limit patients' access to care and place responsibility for health management on individuals.

Stepping back to take a broader look at consumption and medicine in America, archaeology is well positioned to challenge the patient-as-consumer model, despite its dominance in US healthcare policy and contemporary political discourse. Archaeologists have demonstrated how consumer choices are not calibrated equally across the medical field. As Wurst and McGuire (1999) have pointed out, emphasizing "choice" in consumer-choice models implicitly assumes that everyone has unequivocal choice-making opportunities. Consumer behaviors and participation in certain medical marketplaces are limited by patterns of access and structural constraints. Immigrants, women, children, and racialized minorities were expected to meet certain standards of health set by Progressive Era reformers and the professional medical community. This placed an unfair burden on these communities to navigate both economic restraints and a racist and gendered healthcare system. Archaeologists have shown how racialized and gendered social groups navigated healthcare markets to provide care for themselves, but oftentimes in ways that deviated from the expectations of the medical community and pharmaceutical companies. Medicine and health consumer behaviors during the nineteenth and twentieth centuries involved a range of symbolic, economic, and sociopolitical factors. Alternative medicine, in the form of proprietary medicines, offered patients accessible resources and a sanctuary from the professional medical field.

A second, related critique of the patient-consumer model suggests that patients are not consistently able to make educated, informed, and rational decisions regarding their care. Contemporary clinical studies have shown that individuals infrequently make decisions that are best for their well-being in the long run, and that patients are rarely capable of such decisions. People who are sick are often scared, stressed, tired, or unable to make choices. Furthermore, care, defined broadly, is a complex web of social, political, and economic relations. Family members, friends, economic situations, social relationships with doctors and other medical care providers, cultural understandings of health and pharmaceuticals, and patient knowledge interact to create a complex milieu of factors that affect quotidian care-making decisions (Buch 2015).

Rather than a rational process that involves cohesive, sensible choices, healthcare consumption more realistically represents a constant process of "tinkering" (Mol 2008) that is informed by gender ideologies, cultural expectations, and deeply personal affective experiences. In essence, individuals move into and out of patient-hood, but their subjective definitions of what needs to be done (or not done) to be healthy underlie many of their daily practices. Archaeological research supports theories that seek to understand everyday healthcare practices in relation to subjective understandings of health, personal experience, and affective knowledge. Recently, archaeologists have critiqued capitalist paradigms of consumption, arguing that they oversimplify the relationship between consumer choice and self-representation (Cipolla 2017; Creese 2017). By untethering consumption from capitalist consumer-choice models, archaeologists are well poised to examine how affective material relationships engender personal identities and solidify social dependencies (Creese 2017: 63). By closely examining the complex and context-dependent relationships between people and things, Creese (2017) shows how for the Wendat (lower Great Lakes), for example, desire was closely linked to theories of disease. Unfulfilled desires caused mental and physical illness; gifts were essential pharmacopoeia that soothed affective disorders and ensured well-being. Future archaeological research on medical consumerism in capitalist contexts may explore how medicine consumption is also a deeply affective act. Indeed, medicine consumption is an active process that is constrained by patterns of access and informed by subjective health identities and affective relationships (Lee 2017). "Pharmaceuticals and other ingested substances are perhaps the ultimate arena for assessing how value is created through psychological assessments that can outweigh both physical evidence and public external perceptions" (Smith 2007: 421).

Future archaeological research could also explore the affective and subjective qualities of pharmaceutical consumption by focusing on how patent medicine companies undertook a variety of tactics to assert their authority and ensure that patients could easily recognize and use their products. Patent medicine packaging, bottle form, and color fulfilled a "metonymic relationship with [the] contents" (Storm 2018: 59). Since medicine bottles (and their contents) were rarely patented, companies attempted to assuage patient distrust by containing their products in uniquely shaped bottles and branding them with official-sounding text, such as government stamps (Storm 2018: 51). These "tactile signals of authenticity" mitigated consumer fears of adulteration and promoted feelings of trust toward the brand.

Companies also relied on material relationships with medicine vessels and their contents to create intimate, embodied, multisensory experiences. Cues such as medicine's taste, texture, and color appealed to the sensory faculties of patients and lent credibility to the promised cure. While consumers in the early nineteenth century expected a less-than-favorable gustatory experience with patent and proprietary medicines, this came to signal effectiveness: the worse the taste, the better the cure. But mid-nineteenth-century patent medicine manufacturers not only began to make their cures more pleasant tasting, but they also conditioned consumer responses through advertising. For example, Dr. Perregton's Tonic Aperient's "fine aromatic flavour rendered it unequaled as a pleasant and effectual remedy" (*London Standard* 1831; *The Times* 1840). Future archaeological studies might investigate how sensory and metonymical qualities shaped the medical consumer experience and consumption landscape. How did consumers imbue patent medicines with subjective meanings and values? As Smith (2007) notes, individuals who take drugs evaluate them based not only on common knowledge or professional advice, but on what these medications do for them and how they make them feel. How might we evaluate this from an archaeological perspective?

By attending to the social and temporal contexts of medicine use, archaeology shows how health consumption is not a simple, straightforward, or rational decision. Archaeological research opens new horizons for thinking differently about medical patients in America: it demonstrates how patients are constrained by structural and ideological limitations built into the US healthcare system but are also agentive actors who tinker with care strategies to maintain their health.

4

Archaeologies of Public Health

Public health measures mobilized during the COVID-19 crisis, including quarantines, vaccination, and infection tracing, were not recent developments; they were increasingly used in the United States from the eighteenth to twentieth centuries to curb the spread of infectious diseases and improve the overall health of populations. Other public health measures from the same period focused on infrastructure development and urban redesign. European colonization from the seventeenth through nineteenth centuries profoundly altered the disease environment of North America and introduced new ecologies and infectious diseases previously unknown to Native populations. During the nineteenth century, inadequate sewage disposal systems, unclean drinking water, and high population densities in urban areas facilitated the spread of infectious diseases and contributed to high morbidity and mortality rates in the United States (Condran and Crimmins-Gardner 1978: 27). Tuberculosis, typhoid, cholera, measles, influenza, and other infectious disease rates were greatly reduced by the early twentieth century as a result of urban public health measures such as water filtration, improved sewer systems, and disinfection.

Public health is a diverse field of inquiry and practice that includes epidemiology, preventative medicine, and sanitation and infrastructure development. As such, it involves a complex arrangement of assessment measures, methods of intervention, and formal institutions. For the purposes of this chapter, archaeologies of public health will be examined along two axes: bioarchaeological and paleoepidemiological approaches to infectious diseases, and the social politics of public health interventions. Each of these different fields of public health practice incorporates various approaches and practical measures, yet they are often mutually informative. For example, epidemiology, which includes the study of determinants of health and disease (Pearce 1996: 681), is often used to inform the preventative fields of public health. Archaeological research on population health, including research on morbidity and mortality in past populations, infectious disease rates, and preventative public health institutions and practices, follows similar disciplinary boundaries. Historical archaeologists have mobilized bioarchaeological, paleopathological, paleoepidemiological, and material culture-oriented approaches to study population-level health and public health policy and practice in all of their myriad forms.

In archaeology, bioarchaeological, paleopathological, and paleoepidemiological methods have studied rates of infectious disease and illness in past populations. Bioarchaeology, or the study of human remains from archaeological contexts, has often included documenting pathologies in skeletal remains. Within bioarchaeology, biocultural (or life course) approaches have demonstrated the utility of treating skeletal remains as "both biological and cultural" artifacts (Agarwal 2016). These framings stress the importance of long-term (and even multigenerational) environmental and cultural factors to growth, aging, stress, nutrition, activity, and mortality (Zuckerman and Armelagos 2011). The field of paleopathology, in turn, includes the examination and description of physiological disruptions, including illness and mortality, in archaeological populations (Waldron 2017). Paleopathological methods include diagnosing disease presence in human skeletal remains and inferring the frequency, or prevalence, of disease (Waldron 2017). Paleoepidemiology, finally, may be interpreted as an outgrowth of paleopathology: it moves beyond descriptive approaches to interpret determinants of disease in human populations using standardized epidemiological methods (de Souza et al. 2003).

Historical archaeologists working across and within these different subdisciplines have made important contributions by documenting, describing, and explaining patterns of disease and mortality in the past. Paleoepidemiological studies of colonized and enslaved populations, and those that explain the impacts of new disease environments on marginalized social groups, demonstrate the importance of research paradigms that consider social, political, and environmental factors in shaping population health. This is a significant paradigm shift for research on population health, especially for contemporary epidemiological approaches that tend to be mechanistic (focusing on genetic causes) and lean toward individual rather than population scales of analysis (de Souza et al. 2003).

Public health also includes structural interventions that aim to reduce risks to populations, alter social norms to promote public health, and address health problems in ways that are accessible to different social groups. Public health as a preventative practice comprises two biopolitical dimensions: interventions that target health on a population level and policies that target individual health behaviors (what Foucault calls "biopolitics"). Public health includes formal institutions and regulatory measures to mitigate exposure risks and influence the behavior of individuals and populations. These interventions require that public institutions develop frameworks for deciding which populations are deemed contagious, which are most vulnerable, and what practical measures must be taken to mitigate health risks. Social scientists, including historians and archaeologists, have demonstrated that public health exists at the intersection of health technologies and mechanisms of social control. As such, public health is not an apolitical field of practice; social conditions shape one's welfare and well-being, and public health policies, procedures, and institutions are themselves influenced by broader sociopolitical institutions and ideologies. Public health is an inherently political field of practice insofar as it often reifies health inequalities that are linked to specific social identities.

Drawing from historical and archaeological examples, this chapter demonstrates how public health decisions often reinscribe gendered, xenophobic, and racial politics, since public health discourses and practices have historically couched biophysical vulnerability in terms of gender, racial makeup, and citizenship status (Harrison 1994; Krieger 1992, 1999). Archaeological studies show how politicians, reformers, and public health agencies framed contagion and risk in terms of one's gender, age, socioeconomic status, or citizenship status. Historical archaeologists have also shown how public health interventions targeted specific populations considered "at risk" by dint of their gender and citizenship status. At the end of this chapter, I introduce the concept of "biocitizenship" to show how, during the twentieth century, public health was increasingly connected to citizenship status and rights. Biocitizenship can be interpreted as an extension of Foucauldian biopolitics whereby health policy and discourses discipline and control subjects (Happe et al. 2018). Securing the health of populations from infectious disease, such as tuberculosis, became a fulcrum point for broader interpretations of civic belonging and responsibility, as well as gender and domesticity. Public health measures often resulted in a series of material changes to residential housing, foodways, and diet, along with the construction of specialized institutions such as hospitals and asylums.

Finally, as Sontag (2001) argues, illness and health are subjective experiences whose understandings and causalities cannot be divorced from their metaphorical meanings. Some meanings of infectious diseases, like cholera and tuberculosis, are overdetermined insofar as they become "naturalized" in public health discourse and practice. Diseases are imbued with specific metaphorical qualities that are used to promote normative standards of health and express the broader failings of society (Lupton 2012; Wallis and Nerlich 2005). Archaeologies of urban environments and public health demonstrate how immigrants and impoverished communities were often criticized for their poor health and how sickness was frequently framed as a moral failing. As such, health reforms mobilized language that blamed marginalized communities for their own poor health. Historical archaeological studies demonstrate how disease metaphors had material, lasting effects, including the construction of specialized reformatory institutions and the reorganization of urban spaces.

This chapter is organized into four sections. The first section introduces public health and reviews how public health has been defined and studied by social scientists. The second section considers key bioarchaeological methods and interpretive approaches that historical archaeologists have used to study population health. These include bioarchaeological (biocultural), paleopathic, paleoepidemiological, and paleoenvironmental research, using human skeletal remains, ancient pathogens, and parasite remains to address the historic patterns of disease transmission. These methods have provided key insights into the development, application, and sociopolitical effects of public health measures in historic contexts (Milner and Boldsen 2017: 26).

The third section focuses on public health as a form of preventative medicine. The historical archaeological studies in this section demonstrate how preventative health interventions by governments and organizations were entangled in capitalist labor concerns and political philosophies of democratic citizenship. This section also synthesizes social constructivist perspectives that study public health as a site of biopower. These approaches have demonstrated how public health policies were a way of institutionalizing power, monitoring and disciplining populations. Archaeologists have demonstrated how health institutions, including asylums and hospitals, were important for materially and spatially managing the health behaviors of targeted populations.

The fourth section focuses on the social politics of tuberculosis in American public health. Pulmonary tuberculosis, or "consumption," as it was often called, provides one of the most informative and enduring examples of the relationship between disease, power, social inequality, and metaphor. Historians and archaeologists have shown how governments and other organizations employed top-down policies to curb the spread of tuberculosis. These policies included urban restructuring, building specialized medical institutions, and implementing educational programs that encouraged "at risk" populations to modify their choices and behaviors. Here I use the concept of *biocitizenship* to indicate a form of biopolitics meant to manage populations and shape them into better citizens. These public health interventions were tailored by often competing metaphorical, scientific, and sociohistorical understandings of disease (Lupton 1993). These policies also profoundly shaped urban landscapes and altered individuals' material practices and health-seeking behaviors. Archaeological research on tuberculosis institutions reveals how the disease's changing metaphorical qualities had a profound effect on the practical measures taken to contain it, including "moral uplift" and citizenship reform programs that disproportionately targeted women, the working class, and immigrant communities.

What Is Public Health?

Public health includes scientific knowledge, specialized programs, and regulatory agencies focused on maintaining the health of populations (Lupton 1997: 2). It is a heterogeneous field of practice that includes the fields of epidemiology, preventative medicine, sanitation, and infrastructure development. Public health practice also includes analyzing social disparities that shape health inequalities and adopting methods to increase population-level health. Public health requires both healthcare provisions and preventative measures (Lupton 1997). Berridge and colleagues (2011: 6) organize public health along three axes: *health improvement,* which promotes healthy lifestyles and addresses social determinants of health; *health protection,* which protects populations from specific threats, prevents injury, and plans for emergencies; and *health service improvement,* which evaluates health services to ensure effective and safe clinical governance. Health protection frequently targets aggregated populations through environmental infrastructure measures, to include handling wastewater and ensuring general access to safe living conditions (Heller et al. 2003). Health protection operates at both the individual and population level by persuading people to engage in personal hygiene measures and acting to quarantine populations when these proscriptions fail (Porter 2005). Health services include implementing quarantine and vaccination programs to prevent the spread of infectious disease (Rosen 2015).

Public health has the practical goal of assessing mortality and morbidity rates and creating healthier populations by applying information from biomedicine, epidemiology, and genetics (Porter 2005). If public health is "the fulfillment of society's interest in assuring the conditions in which people can be healthy" (Institute of Medicine [US] Committee for the Study of the Future of Public Health 1988: 40), then epidemiology is "the study of the distribution and determinants of disease frequency in human populations" (Savitz 2003: 1151). Epidemiology helps to guide public health, especially by providing rationales for public health policies and by evaluating their effectiveness (Savitz 2003: 1152). Epidemiologists identify the frequencies of chronic and infectious diseases, their causes, and their consequences for population health. These causes need not be strictly biomedical: they may also be social and economic, such as the (in)famous late-twentieth-century discovery regarding the link between smoking tobacco and cancer. Epidemiology can provide scalar approaches to public health management by addressing important determinants of health and disease at the population level and situating them in their social and historical contexts (Pearce 1996: 681).

Finally, public health discourses and policies are always embedded in broader social, political, and economic milieus. As Lupton (1997: 4) notes, "Public health and health promotion are socio-cultural products, [and] their practices, justifications, and logics are subject to change based on political, economic, and other social imperatives." These symbolic and political dimensions have proven fruitful for researchers analyzing how public health discourses and practices have worked to produce certain kinds of subjects (Ayo 2012; Bunton and Petersen 2002; Coveney 1998). Anthropologists and sociologists have shown how public health operates as a site of power and social control, since most modern public health policies are founded on the premise of self-regulation and self-monitoring. As such, health policy and discourse reflect broader sociopolitical debates concerning morality, national belonging, and citizenship (Hosek et al. 2020; Macey 2009). It is also important to note that disciplinary forces are never wholly successful; in other words, they never produce completely docile subjectivities (Thompson 2003). Subjects may resist complying with public health measures entirely or reinterpret public health demands in ways that suit their own perceived needs.

Archaeological Approaches to Public Health

As a discipline that mobilizes method and theory from diverse disciplines, archaeology has successfully bridged the epistemic and ontological divides between epidemiology and public health. Archaeologists are in a unique position to use epidemiological techniques to examine the frequency of specific diseases in the past using human skeletal remains (DeWitte 2016). They also have access to myriad bodies of evidence for conducting research on population health, from pathogens to ancient DNA (aDNA), archival texts, and *materia medica*. Biocultural, paleopathological, and paleoepidemiological research aims to identify the frequency of certain diseases from human remains and identify pathological conditions, while also describing and explaining these patterns in reference to environmental, biomedical, social, and economic causes.

This section discusses how archaeologists have studied public health from bioarchaeological, paleopathological, and paleoepidemiological perspectives. While these approaches differ in their methodologies and theoretical orientations, all use human skeletal remains, ancient pathogens, and parasite remains to address frequencies of chronic and infectious diseases in historic populations and to examine historic patterns of disease transmission. Bioarchaeology and paleopathology use pathogenic indicators on human skeletal remains to study the disease experiences of individuals, while "paleoepidemiology is [also] concerned with documenting past life experience through studies of morbidity and mortality, especially the risks people faced and the means of mitigating them" (Milner and Boldsen 2017: 27). Paleoepidemiological and paleoenvironmental perspectives also demonstrate how social factors, such as economic status, race and gender, and housing arrangements, shaped population-level patterns of morbidity and mortality.

Bioarchaeological (Biocultural) Perspectives

Archaeologists who study population health in the past have frequently done so through bioarchaeological approaches, which include examining human remains for pathological indicators. Within bioarchaeology, bioculturally oriented archaeology moves beyond descriptive analysis to "emphasize the dynamic interaction between humans and their larger social, cultural, and physical environments" (Zuckerman and Armelagos 2011: 20). Biocultural approaches have made significant contributions to studying health and well-being in the past. First, biocultural approaches are multidisciplinary; biocultural research integrates skeletal analysis with archival and material culture studies to examine social, political, and cultural effects on health (Zuckerman and Armelagos 2011). Second, biocultural studies focus on the social determinants of health to interpret the observable physical effects of structural violence and inequality on racialized, gendered, and marginalized social groups (Blakey 2001; Larsen 2002, 2018; Mant et al. 2021; Mant and Holland 2019). These studies have been instrumental to understanding the relationship between social processes and their health impacts on historic populations (Agarwal and Glencross 2011). Finally, biocultural archaeology stresses the importance of the interaction between micro- and global-scale processes in shaping health outcomes (Zuckerman and Armelagos 2011: 20). (A full review of biocultural research is outside the scope of this book, but for comprehensive reviews of health and healthcare in bioarchaeology, see Larsen 2018; Mant and Holland 2019; Tilley and Schrenck 2017.)

Global institutions and their attendant social, economic, and political organizations have impacted the daily lives of individuals on a mass scale. Historical archaeological research on slavery and colonialism has demonstrated how labor regimes and institutionalized racism precipitated extensive demographic changes and poor health outcomes for enslaved and colonized populations (Murphy et al. 2017). European colonization and plantation slavery also stimulated new, previously unknown disease environments as a result of drastic ecological changes (Lightfoot et al. 2013). In North America and the Caribbean, bioarchaeological research on enslaved African and African-descent populations has addressed the physical effects of malnutrition, labor, and inadequate access to healthcare for enslaved people (Blakey 2001; Franklin and Wilson 2020; Shuler 2011). The majority of this work focuses on plantation contexts, although bioarchaeological studies of African diaspora populations have increasingly looked at urban and post-emancipation contexts (Franklin and Wilson 2020). For example, researchers from the African Burial Ground Project in New York determined that enslaved domestic workers in urban settings were subject to similar levels of overwork and malnutrition as enslaved people in plantation settings (Barrett and Blakey 2011; Blakey 2001). This project foregrounds the need for politically and socially situated research by demonstrating how skeletal trauma and malnutrition among enslaved urban populations in New York were the result of structural racism and economic deprivation (Blakey 2001).

Scholars focusing on Native North America have also examined the health impacts of colonization, missionization, and landscape degradation. Researchers concur that European colonization had drastic negative impacts on the health and well-being of Native American people, yet the timing and nature of disease introduction is controversial (Van Buren

2010). Early research into this topic sought to investigate rates of demographic decline as a direct result of the introduction of devastating new diseases, arguing that Indigenous population numbers greatly decreased after Spanish contact (Lovell 1992). But, as Hutchinson (2016) has argued, infectious diseases are not merely biological: they are also social processes that are initiated by human actions and human decisions. Thus, contemporary research has adopted more nuanced approaches to examining health impacts by looking at health status, nutritional status, violence, and cultural change and persistence in more holistic and multidimensional ways (Harrod and Martin 2015; Panich 2013; Stojanowski 2005). Larsen and colleagues' (2001) review of Spanish colonial sites in the Americas uses skeletal stress markers to study the deleterious effects of forced physical labor on Indigenous populations. While all individuals showed signs of physical stress, nutrition, diet, and indicators of interpersonal violence differed across populations. Variability in the health effects of colonization is not surprising, given the cultural and historical specificities of North American Native communities and internal changes to European colonial projects over time. In California and Florida, post-contact dietary changes, especially a decreased reliance on wild game and plants, were concomitant with decreased nutritional health (Walker 2001). In contrast, in the Southwest United States, Puebloan groups suffered higher rates of violence, but they maintained traditional foodways and nutritional behaviors following Spanish colonization (Walker 2001).

Although many archaeologists working with bioarchaeological and paleoepidemiological paradigms have addressed the impacts of European colonization on biological health, fewer studies have specifically addressed health-seeking practices and medicinal systems in the wake of European colonization. Counterexamples include archaeological investigations of Indigenous dwellings at California's Mission Santa Clara de Asís (Panich et al. 2014). The authors integrate ethnohistorical and archaeological data to demonstrate the social complexity of Spanish mission sites and foreground the agency of Indigenous people who resided in these colonial settings. Two bird bone tubes and a large bird of prey talon recovered from the barracks may be related to Yokuts or Ohlone healing practices that continued into the Mission Period (Panich et al. 2014: 482). A large number of tobacco seeds recovered from the barracks also suggest ceremonial use (Panich et al. 2014).

In the Northeast US, archaeological research has focused on sartorial expressions and how they exemplified power and meaning within Native societies—including in contexts of well-being (Bragdon 2017). The adoption of ready-made European clothing and cloth by Native people in post-contact periods was not merely determined by patterns of access; "techniques of the body" referenced broader ideas about disease and health (Bragdon 2017). Wearing European textiles may have "added another 'protective' layer" from infectious (European) diseases (Bragdon 2017: 122). Creese (2017) similarly investigates the changing socialization of objects, in this case clay smoking pipes, among the Wendat (or Huron) during the seventeenth century. In this context, objects, especially those associated with the body, undertook important "emotion work" (Creese 2017). Specific pipe effigies may have been associated with healing and aimed to promote emotional and physical well-being. Pipe use increased in the 1630s and 1640s, coinciding with European-introduced epidemics.

While bioarchaeological and paleoepidemiological research has provided a great deal of information regarding the timing, prevalence, and biological effects of epidemic infectious diseases on Native populations, more object-focused research like that mentioned previously is needed to acquire a nuanced understanding of the social-material and health-related practices associated with new disease environments.

Paleoepidemiological Perspectives

In the nineteenth and twentieth centuries, well-known epidemiologists, such as John Snow and John Graunt, developed statistical standards for examining disease prevalence within specific populations (Pearce 1996). These methods have been refined through developments in research design and modern data-analysis techniques (Pearce 1996: 679). More recent developments in epidemiology have attended a shift in the scale of analysis from the population to the individual. Genomic advances, in particular, have altered the scope and purpose of epidemiology by focusing on individuals and cohorts who are similarly affected by genetic variances. Recent calls for more holistic paradigms in epidemiology stress the need for multidisciplinary approaches that account for social, economic, and biological determinants of health (Pearce 1996: 680). This includes considering epigenetic factors as well as examining how systemic inequalities affect population morbidity and mortality.

Paleoepidemiology, like contemporary epidemiology, attempts to determine rates of morbidity and mortality based on the presence of specific disease etiologies (Waldron 2017). Paleoepidemiological research in historical archaeology has focused on examining infectious diseases and their consequences via the study of human skeletal remains and their pathogenic indicators. Paleoepidemiologists address patterns of trauma, chronic disease, and infectious disease in populations by analyzing the presence of pathologies, such as skeletal lesions and tooth abnormalities. This work aims to reconstruct the spatial, temporal, and social distribution of health and disease in past populations (Waldron 2017). Infectious diseases in humans are caused by a range of pathogenic agents, including bacteria, viruses, protozoa, and worms (Larsen 2018: 296). Different pathogens produce different morbidity and mortality profiles, ranging from chronic sickness to death, and they may be endemic or epidemic within a population. As Mitchell (2003) notes, the reproductive success of pathogens in humans is contingent upon their introduction to concentrated communities in densely populated, often unsanitary conditions, and the quick, geographically expansive mobility of their hosts (Mitchell 2003: 172).

Paleoepidemiology is a multidisciplinary subfield that integrates methods and theories from bioarchaeology, paleopathology, and molecular biology to reconstruct past conditions of disease in populations in reference to lifestyle and environment (de Souza et al. 2003). Like epidemiologists, paleoepidemiologists analyze the distribution and frequency of disease in specified populations, but their research questions and outcomes are constrained to specific time periods and incomplete archaeological data (de Souza et al. 2003). Much paleoepidemiological research focuses on the frequency, spatial distribution, and health impacts of infectious disease. Infectious disease has been a consistent part of the human experience for millennia, but its effects and human attempts to mitigate them have changed across temporal and geographic scales (Mitchell 2003: 171). Historical archaeological research has identified the presence of infectious disease and comorbidities in past populations and has addressed social determinants of health and disease. Despite some contemporary scholars' claims that epidemics (particularly pandemics) act as social levelers (Scheidel 2018), infectious diseases often exacerbate preexisting structural inequalities (Bowleg 2020). They disproportionately affect already precarious populations (Abedi et al. 2021; Patel et al. 2020). They also throw into broad relief structural inequalities in health provision systems, the poor health outcomes of those with inadequate access to care, and vulnerabilities in employment, housing, food, and water supplies (Armelagos et al. 2005; Farmer 1996).

Because of their access to human skeletal remains, ancient pathogens, and material culture, archaeologists are well positioned to study the disease experiences of individuals and identify the public health measures that populations took to mitigate the harm caused by infectious diseases (DeWitte 2016). As archaeologists have argued, infectious diseases in humans are inseparable from their social consequences, whether in terms of declining demographic rates, practical measures used to alleviate the effects of disease, or the social-metaphorical qualities that are inscribed on the bodies of those who suffer (Larsen 2018; Mitchell 2003; Roberts and Manchester 2010). Infectious diseases commonly affect soft tissues, such as organs, skin, and muscles, and thus may not be identifiable in human skeletal material alone (Martin et al. 2013). Furthermore, as evidence, skeletal lesions are often inconclusive; they may be caused by different factors, including nutritional deficiencies, physical stress, and chronic disease, in addition to pathogenic infections (Larsen 2018). Because of these complicating factors, paleoepidemiologists often use multiple lines of evidence (such as historical records and paleoenvironmental evidence) to investigate disease impact.

Paleoepidemiological approaches to infectious diseases have shown how prior to the Columbian Exchange, which precipitated the spread of pathogens and hosts on an unprecedented global scale, human societies were impacted by new pathogenic environments as a result of their changing relationships with plant and animal communities (Bendrey and Martin 2021; Fournié et al. 2017). Plant and animal domestication, a process that roughly dates to 10,000 years before present, and anthropogenic landscape changes precipitated the introduction of zoonotic diseases to human communities (Mitchell 2003). Examples include cholera infections caused by animal feces contamination and high rates of malaria in agricultural settings where standing water was present (for a comprehensive review, see Bendrey and Martin 2021).

By the fifteenth century, European colonialism was facilitating new ecologies of disease (Porter 2005: 46). This so-called second epidemiological transition is marked by the Industrial Revolution in the West (Zuckerman, Harper et al. 2014). New labor regimes, mechanization, and urban population density significantly altered the disease landscape in America, presenting new challenges for public health. Infectious diseases predominately affected populations who were vulnerable, such as those with limited access to adequate sanitation, clean water, nutrition, and healthcare (Roberts 2020). Epidemics brought from Europe, including smallpox, mumps, measles, and scarlet fever, had devastating impacts on both Indigenous and urbanized societies throughout the Atlantic region. As archaeologists and historians have argued, the so-called Columbian Exchange not only triggered the global transfer of people, plants, animals, and ideas, but also introduced infectious diseases, transformed ecosystems, and significantly altered floral and faunal populations (Cameron et al. 2015; Hutchinson 2016; Lightfoot et al. 2013).

Paleoenvironmental Perspectives

New developments in ancient pathogen genomic research and parasitology have greatly aided paleoenvironmental approaches to health. Both fields specifically examine disease carriers, including viruses, parasites, and pathogens. Those found at archaeological sites provide direct evidence regarding past disease environments and indirect evidence of the health status of human populations. Much historical archaeological research on pathogenic environments includes vertebrate and invertebrate zoology in the investigation of disease hosts (Fisher et al. 2007; Hufthammer and Walløe 2013; Reinhard 1992, 2017); pathogen genomic research (Duchêne et al. 2020); and paleobotany and palynology for reconstructing past environmental conditions (Bryant and Holloway 1983; Dincauze 2000). Archaeological parasitology is the study of parasite distribution; this helps to develop detailed analyses of the dietary, medicinal, and environmental factors that shaped patterns of infection (Reinhard 2017). Pathoecology, or the study of parasitism in its cultural and environmental context (Reinhard et al. 2013), has offered nuanced insights into public health and infectious disease. Parasites and parasite eggs recovered from sensitive cultural contexts, such as privies, provide incontrovertible evidence of infection in human populations (Reinhard 2017). Parasites also provide information on past pathogenic environments.

As Fisher and colleagues (2007) argue, humans constantly alter their environments and must adapt to the health conditions that these environmental changes precipitate. Archaeological research in Albany, New York, by Fisher and colleagues (2007) indicates that urban populations were exposed to a host of different parasitic infections throughout the nineteenth century. Abundance measures of parasite eggs, recovered from household latrines in Albany, suggest that parasite numbers increased significantly in conjunction with the expansion of human populations in the late eighteenth century. Archaeological samples from privies indicate the presence of louse nits, roundworms, pinworms, whipworms, and tapeworms (Fisher et al. 2007). Sanitary planning activities during the 1850s and 1860s, such as enclosing sewage systems, controlling seepage, and carrying fresh water into the city from reservoirs, helped to curb the spread of parasites (Fisher et al. 2007). Archaeological examples such as these demonstrate the value of parasitology research for examining past disease environments, as well as studying the effectiveness of public health measures in abating diseases.

Archaeologies of Public Health from Material Culture Perspectives

In addition to examining human skeletal remains and ancient pathogenic environments, historical archaeologists use material culture to interpret treatments and preventative strategies to manage health in the past. These material culture-oriented approaches fall into two general categories. One body of research focuses on public health as preventative medicine. This work examines disease-prevention methods adopted by institutions and organizations, or what may be called the "science and art of preventing disease" (Winslow 1920). These include workplace health campaigns, public sanitation programs, and urban restructuring and spatial reorganization. Archaeologists have demonstrated how these programs to mitigate public health risks often intersected with capitalist values concerning wage labor and profit maximization. The other vein of archaeological research demonstrates how public health references broad networks of social relations and mobilizes disease metaphors that entrench unequal relations of power. This vein may be called "social constructivist" insofar as it exposes the ways in which scientific categories and systems of knowledge about the body and health become naturalized through public health policy. This knowledge also produces certain kinds of material practices. The following sections will detail both of these methodological and interpretive approaches.

Public Health as Preventative Medicine: Workplace Health

As a branch of preventative medicine, public health has a long global history; health policies and practices existed in urban contexts in Assyria, Mesopotamia, Greece, and Rome (Porter 2005: 13). Ancient public health systems relied on practical measures to ensure healthful environments. These measures included street planning, ensuring access to clean drinking water, and managing bodily waste (Rosen 2015). Differing theories also foregrounded the management of food, water, air, and animals for abating the spread of contagious disease (Porter 2005: 13). In this sense, public health was a matter of both controlling individual bodies and managing environmental conditions to mitigate exposures to harmful substances. Hippocratic medical practice and theory, though originally dating to the early half of the first century AD, was practiced throughout Europe and its colonies until the late eighteenth century. Euro-American medical science was not based in scientific practice (involving hypothesis testing and experimentation) until the late nineteenth century (Porter 2005; Rosen 2015). Instead, Hippocratic theories concerning bodily humors and environmental determinism, or "medical meteorology," shaped the field of public health in Europe and the United States until the development of post-Enlightenment bacteriology and clinical science in the nineteenth century (Rosen 2015).

Mirroring intellectual and scientific trends in European countries, public health interventions in the United States during the nineteenth century were often embedded in broader economic concerns. During this period, state governments and private companies adopted public health measures to ensure the health and productivity of American workforces. These measures included private health insurance options, which could be purchased from one's employer, and workplace health programs. The idea that health was paramount to capitalist gains has its roots in eighteenth-century administration models, particularly cameralism (Rosen 1953). This was a sixteenth-century political philosophy of the Habsburg Empire, which viewed the role of the government as the protector of the general populace (Porter 2005: 53). In eighteenth-century Germany, the government considered a growing and healthy population to be a significant source of national strength in terms of expanding agricultural, military, and industrial power. Medical police, or *policey,* emerged in Germany as a civil administrative taskforce to ensure the state's social welfare (Porter 2005: 53; Rosen 1953). Medical police were tasked with supervising pharmacy practice, enforcing medical licensing, and standardizing medical fees and associated costs (Rosen 1953). In Sweden, state health programs performed targeted measures aimed at increasing population growth through hygiene and fertility education, abating sexually transmitted diseases, and developing municipal hospitals (Porter 2005: 54). In France, collective health administration was ill-regarded in the postrevolutionary period, but in 1791 a health committee was developed under the state's aegis to establish a network of rural health officers (Porter 2005: 57).

In North America, state-administered public health programs were decentralized until the eighteenth century, when citizens' health became a primary concern for employers, physicians, city planners, and civic reformers (Berridge et al. 2011). The growth of public health as a field of study and practice paralleled the rise of centralized government agencies in the United States (Porter 2005: 49). For American civic reformers and government agencies, population-level health was essential to a wealthy, successful nation. Methods for assessing the political strength of the nation by counting healthy members of the population were popularized by the English scientist William Petty (Porter 2005: 49). These methods were adopted by American public health agencies and institutions. Petty argued that the strength of the physical body and the aptitude of the nation (or the body politic) were intrinsically connected. During the eighteenth century in Britain, official discourses on public health were infused with capitalist ideologies. In the United States, government agencies and policymakers viewed the productive capacities of workers as essential to the success of wage labor, ensuring a steady flow of income. It was through successfully performing "health" that both the working class and capitalists could gauge success in the new capitalist world order (Porter 2005). As Foucault notes, administrative concerns for the well-being of populations were grounded in managing the economic productivity of individual bodies.

During the nineteenth century, private companies adopted many of the government agencies' health concerns. Protecting the health of one's labor force was paramount to capitalist accumulation. Historical archaeological research has shown how capitalist values concerning employment and health affected laboring populations in nineteenth-century America. One example is Carley's (1981) archaeological research at Fort Vancouver, Washington, established by the Hudson Bay Company as a fur trading post in 1824–1825 (Carley 1981: 19). At Fort Vancouver, epidemic fevers (likely malaria) occurred throughout the 1820s and 1830s. These fever outbreaks negatively impacted the fort's labor force since employees would be sick for days or weeks at a time (Carley 1981: 33). Records indicate that company doctors used a range of "heroic" treatment methods to treat sick workers, including venesection and administering quinine for fevers. Archaeological excavations at the Riverside Complex, which included domestic quarters and the company hospital, uncovered medicine bottles, cupping devices, and liquor bottles. Researchers also excavated large "smoking" pits that may have been used to purify the air of bad miasmas during fever outbreaks. Public health measures, such as the firepits and the company hospital, along with personal care practices on the part of company employees, demonstrate the degree to which the Hudson Bay Company was invested in maintaining its workforce's health (Carley 1981).

Similar archaeological research at Butt Valley, California, provides evidence of company policies regarding health and sanitation. During the early 1900s, the urban demand for safe drinking water spurred the construction of massive dams, reservoirs, and aqueduct systems across the western United States (Maniery 2002: 69). These construction efforts necessitated the development of worker camps designed to organize, service, and house thousands of dam employees. From 1901–1924, the Great Western Power (GWP) Company completed a series of dam projects in Butt Valley. Over the years, a series of residential houses, cookhouses, bathhouses, and hospitals were built in the area. In 1913, the state passed the California Labor Camp Sanitation Act to protect laborers from poor living and working conditions. Sanitation Act measures and regulations included requirements for clean drinking water, proper sewage systems, a healthful diet, and a clean living space for all employees. Targeted analysis of architectural features and artifacts recovered from the camp indicate that GWP took pains to follow state and federal sanitation and hygiene guidelines in order to maximize the health (and laboring capacity) of employees (Maniery 2002). As these examples demonstrate, practical sanitation reforms were a form of capital, since implementing them could secure the health and productive output of company workers.

Public Health as Preventative Medicine: Urban Restructuring and Public Health Infrastructure

Other archaeological studies explore the power-laden ideological underpinnings of preventative health projects and how public health ideologies affect infrastructure and urban planning. Much of this work focuses on the relationships between infectious disease, infrastructure development, urban planning, and housing reform in urban areas, given that cities have long been targeted by social reformers (Fisher et al. 2007). These archaeological studies integrate diverse lines of evidence, such as written documents, material culture, and bioarchaeology, to investigate the health impacts on urban communities of drinking water and sewage projects, neighborhood restructuring, and housing reforms (Beisaw 2016; Betsinger and DeWitte 2020; Howson 1993). Infectious diseases, particularly cholera, malaria, and yellow fever, were prevalent in urban areas during the nineteenth and early twentieth centuries and incentivized burgeoning city health departments to restructure housing, drinking water, and sewage systems (Howson 1993: 143). As a densely populated urban area, New York in particular has yielded important archaeological data on these topics, given the city's long history of dense population, immigration, public health initiatives, and numerous development projects.

Werner and Novak's (2010) research in New York mobilizes Foucault's work on bodily discipline and the idea of the "body-city nexus" to explore the relationships between health, disease, and civic authority in the nineteenth century. As the authors argue, social and political relations shape medical knowledge (Werner and Novak 2010). Medical knowledge serves to monitor and regulate the bodies of citizens to ensure good health and productivity, while also differentiating between specific social groups. Werner and Novak's (2010) research traces how authoritative discourses regarding biological difference, moral and religious authority, and mid-nineteenth-century sanitation policies authorized the spatial segregation of certain social groups. The authors integrate bioarchaeological, material culture, and archival analyses to study the lives of individuals interred within the Spring Street Presbyterian Church in New York (1811–1840s). Indicators of physical labor and poor living conditions were present on many of the skeletal remains. These included robust muscle attachments, evidence of trauma, lesions on bones indicating tuberculosis infections, and lesions associated with congenital and venereal syphilis. By the 1830s, city officials had initiated citywide public health measures to encourage social uplift among the poorer classes by providing them with clean drinking water and sewers; they also monitored citizens' behavior via a series of fire/police watchtowers (Werner and Novak 2010: 111). The authors ultimately demonstrate the usefulness of archaeological research in elucidating how material manifestations of public health reform, civic order, and sanitary projects articulate with individual understandings of citizenship and health. They conclude that sanitary reform measures exemplified new power relationships that fed into theories of race and class, which naturalized the inadequate living conditions and poor health outcomes of Spring Street residents.

A study by Howson (1993), also in New York, similarly addresses public health, sanitation, and access to healthcare resources in households in Greenwich Village. This research focuses on artifacts recovered from nineteenth- to early twentieth-century cisterns and privies in Washington Square (Howson 1993). Population growth during the early 1800s precipitated suburban spread to Greenwich Village. Differences in household cistern and privy abandonment dates (1830s-1870s) indicate that wealthier households were the first to adopt indoor plumbing, although attitudes toward it were ambivalent across social classes (Howson 1993: 142).

Nineteenth-century citizens' attitudes toward water closets and sewers were paradoxical: they were at once desired and affordable among middle- and middle-upper-class households but were also deemed dangerous due to the sewer gases and dangerous miasmas that escaped them. In this light, the sanitation movement in New York illustrates the nineteenth-century relationships between science, technology, and urban culture. Miasmic theories of contagion (and later germ theory) replaced older theories that viewed diseases as "fostered by moral shortcomings of the poor" (Howson 1993: 143). Changing attitudes toward public health and the increased availability of sanitary material culture, such as water closets, led to a demand for practical domestic solutions to public health problems across all social classes. Finally, as Stottman (2000) argues, privies are an invaluable form of material culture for revealing perceptions of sanitation. Vault depth, materials, methods of construction, and proximity to drinking water sources all provide indispensable information concerning people's understanding of sanitation and health (Stottman 2000).

Other archaeological studies of public health and urbanization in New York have focused on the infamous neighborhood of Five Points (Figure 4.1). Historical archaeologists have examined the lived experiences of residents in the neighborhood, many of whom suffered from work-related trauma, infectious diseases, and unsanitary living conditions (Bonasera and Raymer 2001; Cantwell and Wall 2001; Fitts 2001; Yamin 1998). Originally established as a preindustrial, middle-class, residential neighborhood in the early 1700s, Five Points later developed into a crowded urban space (Yamin 1998). Municipal sanitary legislation outlawing the operation of "miasmic producing" industries within the residential areas drew slaughterhouses and industrial processing plants to the "Collect," a once-middle-class area of the city. In 1802, the city's Health Office suggested filling in the Collect to mitigate the spread of dangerous infectious diseases, such as yellow fever. Alas, the fill was unstable, toxic, and full of dangerous "miasmas," resulting in middle-class residents fleeing from the area. By the 1830s, Five Points was once again inhabited by free Black communities, Irish immigrants, and working-class families (Yamin 1998). Despite city sanitation and public health reforms, archaeologies of Five Points demonstrate how racialized and poor communities have disproportionately been the subjects of development projects. But, historically, sanitation reform has still not mitigated the ill health effects of environmental pollution for marginalized communities.

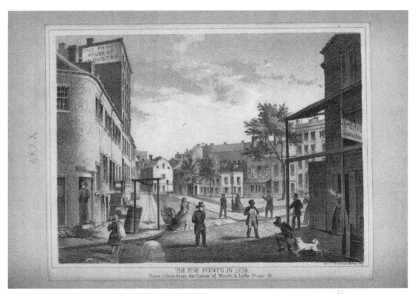

Figure 4.1. Five Points, New York, 1859. Lithograph for *D.T. Valentine's Manual*, 1860. Wikimedia Commons, public domain.

Key to the success of urban infrastructure projects was the ability to represent and organize space through mapping. Mapping "at risk" populations via cartographic projects entailed identifying environmental risks that were often then associated with poverty. Mapping was a key technique for tracing the spatial contours of epidemics and delineating the boundaries of diseased spaces. One of the most well-known examples of medical mapping is John Snow's trace mapping of a cholera outbreak in London in 1854 (McLeod 2000). Snow's medical mapping techniques set a precedent for public health policy and governmental oversight, as nineteenth-century maps were used to demarcate diseased bodies, pockets of disorder, overpopulation, and working-class vice and disease (Gilbert 2004).

Historians and archaeologists working on public health infrastructure have adopted critical approaches to the relationships between disease, race, marginalization, and urban space (Craddock 1995, 1998). For example, Craddock (2000) explores the coproduction of race, place, and pathology in nineteenth-century San Francisco, California. Craddock shows how disease and depravity were mapped onto the bodies of Chinese Americans in Chinatown, San Francisco. Immigrants, the poor, the working classes, and people of color have overwhelmingly been framed as both the victims and the perpetrators of communicable disease, while "their" spaces, to include houses, neighborhoods, and schools, are frequently viewed by policymakers as sites of contagion and infection (Allen 2008; Craddock 1999). As Craddock (1995: 958) argues, any examination of infectious disease must include the ways that diseases are spatially defined and controlled "through metaphoric associations of place and affliction, inscriptions of contagious space, and the restructuring of purportedly diseased environments." The fusion of place and disease in public health is well documented in historical and geographic research, particularly in urban and colonial contexts, where the relationship between space and the "other" worked to geographically delineate social difference along racial, economic, and gendered lines (Anderson 2006; Brown and Duncan 2002; Craddock 1998; Peterson 1979).

Warner-Smith's (2020) work investigates the various ways that cholera epidemics in the Caribbean were spatialized by what she calls "cholera narratives." Warner-Smith's research draws from postcolonial scholarship, critical geography, and archaeology to show how maps act as an instrument of authoritative state power but can also allow for local understandings of epidemics. Local maps of cholera in the Caribbean outline how outbreaks on the islands were experienced and interpreted at different regional scales (Warner-Smith 2020). This study demonstrates how cartography is both restraining and generative; spatial practices and representations are used as tools of the state, but they can simultaneously illuminate micro-scale, subjective experiences of space.

Public Health as a Site of Biopower: Social Constructivist Approaches

Public health definitions change throughout time, and these temporal changes reflect different historical configurations of health, the individual, responsibility, and choice. In the late 1800s, new advancements in bacteriology and epidemiology influenced the scope and direction of public health policies (Porter 2005). After the urban reform and environmental movements of the early 1800s, Progressive Era public health organizations aimed to improve people's lives through individual "lifestyle changes" (Hoy 1997; Smith 2008). Instead of focusing on sweeping infrastructure and sanitary reforms, public health took on a new role: directing individual behavior. Health optimization programs included information about the importance of education, exercise, and healthful eating, abstaining from alcohol and drugs, and refraining from "immoral" sexual behaviors (Lupton 1997).

Under the aegis of the "new public health" (Lupton 1997), individuals were discouraged from participating in risky activities while also being encouraged to seek resources, such as preventative medicines, that could increase their well-being.

This shift in public health policy from state and federal responsibility to individual/civic responsibility mirrored broader social attitudes in the United States concerning the role of the state and individual accountability. Victorian-era reform movements (1890–1920s) sought to place the onus of good health on individuals and families; the responsibility of government agencies and reformatory institutions was to instill in individuals a preoccupation with health-enhancing activities through personal lifestyle decisions. This early twentieth-century ethos of individual responsibility and anti-government intervention came to a head in the 1980s, when neoliberal governance within the United States during the Reagan administration similarly spurred the deregulation and privatization of public health services. This more recent "new" public health was likewise informed by neoliberal political and social trends that increasingly focused on individual responsibility and choice. It has had lasting repercussions in terms of burgeoning health inequalities and imbalanced access to care for minority populations (Petersen and Lupton 1996).

Social scientists who study the changing landscape of public health and policy have found Michel Foucault's work particularly helpful in thinking about power and authority. Foucault represents one of the most oft-cited scholars interested in critiquing the ways that people in positions of power mobilize knowledge and scientific concepts. By deconstructing, or tracing the historical genealogies of, specific categories (such as illness, homosexuality, and insanity), Foucault demonstrated that these taken-for-granted classifications are socially constructed through discourses concomitant with the emergence of new authorities and institutions. Health categories such as normality, risk, and health rely on authoritative commands to knowledge that obscure the conditional nature of these categories. For constructivist scholars, categories in public health are guided by an ontological reality but are "true" because they develop within a complex nexus of power.

One of the most potent moves by the modern state was the "emergence of the health and physical well-being of the population in general as one of the essential objectives of political power" (Foucault et al. 1997: 94). Foucault outlines two dimensions of "biopower" that describe the way political power works (Cisney and Morar 2016). The first form of biopower is exercised on the individual body, while the second dimension of power works through the body politic. Managing the individual body and body politic requires institutions, including schools, hospitals, asylums, and sanatoria. Institutions are brought into existence by society's need to manage, supervise, or otherwise control aspects of social life, including medicine and public health. Foucault argues that nonnormative bodies can be consigned to institutions to be monitored or punished, which entails techniques of the body and material interventions (Bevir 1999).

Foucault's influence on historical archaeologists interested in public health have led them to focus on regulatory institutions such as plantations (Delle 1998; Orser 1990; Singleton 1995), missions (Graham 1998; Panich and Schneider 2015), schools (Gibb and Beisaw 2000), almshouses (Spencer-Wood 2001), prisons (Casella 2000), and asylums (Spencer-Wood and Baugher 2001). Fundamental questions in this research include: What is an institution? How do institutions work? What are the individual and collective effects of institutionalization? Archaeologists have argued that institutions sought to establish predictable behavior across multiple sectors of society (De Cunzo 2006). "Total institutions" are extreme examples of attempts to modify behavior through strict, all-encompassing forms of regulation and punishment (Baugher 2009). Archaeological studies of total institutions include work on prisons, reformatories, and penitentiaries (Casella 2000, 2007; Sutton 2003). Transformative institutions, such as schools, almshouses, and clinics, sought to alter the behaviors, beliefs, habits, and lifestyles of gendered, racialized, and ethnic minorities. These institutions perpetuated normative behavioral concepts and theories regarding the perceived moral and physical failings of marginalized social groups (De Cunzo 2006). Medical institutions, including hospitals and sanatoria, perpetuated narrow definitions of morality (according to the dominant classes), which affected how physical nonnormativity, poverty, and nonnormative family structures were interpreted (De Cunzo 2006: 207).

Archaeologists have approached institutions via two related interpretive lenses. The first concerns the modes of social control that certain institutions adopted to transform noncompliant, pathologized, and otherwise nonnormative subjects of the state into productive citizens. During the eighteenth century, influxes of immigrants and a rise in what was considered the "able-bodied poor" led to the development of reformatory institutions, including almshouses, poorhouses, and reformatories themselves

(De Cunzo 1995). These institutions contained populations who were to be educated out of their own indigence through hard work, temperance, and cleanliness (Lans 2022). Archaeologists have addressed the various mechanisms (rhetorical, spatial, material) mobilized by institutions to transform people's daily existence, including the ways they ate, worked, clothed themselves, participated in public and political life, and engaged in social and sexual relationships (Beisaw and Gibb 2009). This research invariably draws on Foucault's work on sexuality, discipline, and biopolitics to address questions related to social identities, such as class, gender, race, ethnicity, and sexuality, and how these intersected with organizational goals and moral attitudes. Archaeologies of charitable institutions, including almshouses and hospitals, have shown how authorities' ideals concerning family structures, behavior, and physical normativity were linked to the moral aptitudes of their patients (De Cunzo 2006). While charitable institutions were ostensibly designed to care for the less fortunate, they also sought to reform residents through restrictions on dress, diet, and sociality—for if poverty and disease were symptoms of one's moral deficiency, then one could be uplifted through a strict regimen (Baugher 2009).

The second vein of research on institutions has explored the degree to which mechanisms of control were successful and how affected individuals resisted dominant modes of power. Archaeological and archival research at the Magdalen Society of Philadelphia, for example, shows how this institution for "fallen women" perpetuated normative working-class and gendered values, though inmates often negotiated their roles as domestic workers in training (De Cunzo 1995). Female convicts and factory workers in prisons in Australia similarly renegotiated normative ascriptions of gender, sexuality, and motherhood in their material practices (Casella 2000).

Other sites of control and resistance include asylums and state hospitals. Both were designed to house individuals who were officially considered difficult or "insane." Definitions of mental illness changed throughout the course of the nineteenth and early twentieth centuries, and "deviant" behaviors were variously interpreted as inherited from family members or as rooted in one's immoral nature (Psota 2011: 22). Asylums were institutions developed by medical professionals during the nineteenth and twentieth centuries to provide housing, care, and treatment for mentally ill patients. Asylums were meant to physically isolate mentally ill individuals from the broader society and relieve families of caretaking duties (Psota 2011). Historical documents, court records, firsthand accounts, and material culture related to asylums overwhelmingly indicate that staff and doctors were frequently abusive and injurious toward their patients. Most families viewed asylums as a last resort, accessed only when they were no longer physically or financially able to care for family members. Examination of objects recovered from an early twentieth-century household in San Jose, California, illustrates the complex intersections between at-home care and institutionalization for one family (Psota 2011). Archaeological material recovered from the Finger/Sengstacken household includes an array of hygiene products, patent medicine bottles, and unlabeled pharmacy bottles, which show how family members coped with caring for a loved one. Psota concludes that the unmarked bottles likely contained medication for treating the residents' daughter, Tillie, who was diagnosed with mental illness at an early age. Given the long and public histories of abuse and mistreatment by Bay Area institutions, it is likely that family members preferred to care for Tillie at home. She was eventually institutionalized at Agnews State Hospital in Stockton, California, where she died from sepsis at the age of forty-three.

Case Study: Tuberculosis

The remainder of this chapter focuses on pulmonary tuberculosis, or "consumption," as it was frequently called during the nineteenth century. Tuberculosis provides an abiding example of the complex, and often conflicting, web of ideologies, meanings, and public health measures associated with disease. Exploring the social history of tuberculosis necessitates touching upon themes previously discussed in this chapter, including sanitation, urban and spatial design, the development of public hospitals and asylums, and the potency of disease metaphors. Perhaps because of the significant impact of this disease on US mortality and morbidity rates, or because of the profound social meanings that have been attached to the disease over the past 200 years, tuberculosis remains one of the most often studied infectious diseases in clinical medicine, medical history, and archaeology. Early medical historical accounts of tuberculosis adopted top-down approaches that focused on the progression of medical science in disease etiology, diagnosis, and treatment, and characterized the physicians and scientists who were essential to key developments in medicine, policy, and public health (Condrau 2010). More recently, historians have adopted micro-scale approaches to the history of tuberculosis, detailing tuberculosis patients' experiences in relationship to social, political, and scientific settings (Bates 1992).

Archaeological approaches to tuberculosis have undergone similar theoretical and methodological evolutions. Bioarchaeological and paleoepidemiological studies have made invaluable contributions to understanding the timing and emergence of tuberculosis among prehistoric and historic populations. Despite these important inroads, the presence or absence of disease does not necessarily provide detailed information about individual or group experiences of illness, nor does it automatically demonstrate broader social meanings (Condrau 2010). Given the limitations of biological approaches, historical archaeologists have drawn from diverse social theories to examine the larger social and political ideologies that were entangled with tuberculosis. Archaeologists have also used multiple forms of evidence, including historical documents, literary texts, and material culture, to study the enduring relationship between disease, power and social inequality, and metaphor. As Sontag (2001) reminds us, illness is always interpreted through a social lens, and it acquires specific metaphorical associations that shape disease etiologies, treatments, and social perceptions. And as proponents of embodiment theory have pointed out, human health and physiology cannot be divorced from multiscalar social processes such as power, agency, violence, and marginalization (Scheper-Hughes and Lock 1987; Sheridan and Gregoricka 2020; Tung 2021).

The metaphorical and ideological qualities imbued in tuberculosis had lasting material effects for large swaths of the American population, especially for women, urban residents, and immigrant communities. Responses to tuberculosis on the part of medical organizations, city planners, and health reformers helped to reshape urban topographies. Agencies and organizations also initiated the construction of specialized establishments, such as state hospitals and sanatoria, to cure and isolate patients. Healthcare in these institutions often targeted residents' symptoms through moral reform meant to instill civic values in patients. Finally, tuberculosis was imbued with ideological traits that connected the disease to morality, gender, and citizenship.

Etiologies and Symptoms of Tuberculosis

Tuberculosis is an infectious disease caused by two species of *Mycobacterium: Mycobacterium tuberculosis* and *Mycobacterium bovis* (Larsen 2018; Roberts and Buikstra 2003). Pulmonary tuberculosis, which makes up 90 percent of cases, involves infections of the lungs and pulmonary system. Extrapulmonary tuberculosis, in which infection spreads outside of the lungs to other parts of the body, is far less common. Tuberculosis typically includes diagnostic symptoms such as fever, decreased appetite, and coughing (Roberts and Buikstra 2003). Risk factors for tuberculosis include smoking, vitamin D deficiency, infection with HIV, close contact with animals, and living or working in overcrowded conditions (Narasimhan et al. 2013; Roberts 2020). Today, non-antibiotic-resistant strains of tuberculosis may be treated using courses of multiple antibiotics. Historically, before the widespread use of antibiotics, tuberculosis was chronic and/or fatal. The disease is often concurrent with vitamin D–related ailments, to include rickets and osteomalacia, and tuberculosis infection rates are higher in people who are not exposed to sufficient levels of UV light (Narasimhan et al. 2013).

Bioarchaeological evidence for tuberculosis exists for European and pre-Columbian North American contexts. The timing and origins of tuberculosis are contested. Archaeologists have assumed that *M. tuberculosis* emerged in Europe and Western Asia during Neolithic periods when human communities were in contact with cattle and *M. bovis* (Buzic and Giuffra 2020; Larsen 2018). Molecular and osteological research indicates that strains of *M. tuberculosis* were also present in the precontact Americas, for example as demonstrated by the presence of the disease in skeletal samples from Chile and Peru (Larsen 2018). However, molecular genetic research indicates that strains of *M. tuberculosis* are similar in Europe and the Americas, suggesting that Old World strains replaced precontact New World strains. Archaeological and historical evidence indicates that during the eighteenth and nineteenth centuries, industrialization and urbanization, increased factory work and exposure to particulate pollution, and crowded living conditions resulted in high tuberculosis rates across North America and Europe (Roberts 2020).

Skeletal lesions consistent with clinical cases of tuberculosis may manifest months to years after initial infection, thus enabling osteological identification of the disease (Larsen 2018). Unfortunately, bone changes in tuberculosis patients are rare and 3–7 percent of skeletal indicators are nonspecific (Roberts and Buikstra 2003). The most reliable osteological indicator of tuberculosis infection is lesions on the thoracis and lumbar vertebrae, while diagnosis based on bone lesions throughout the rest of the body is more tentative (Roberts and Buikstra 2003). Possible indicators include osteomyelitis on joints and periosteal lesions on the ribs and long bones (Cooper et al. 2016; Roberts and Buikstra 2003). Other paleopathological methods for tuberculosis diagnosis in archaeological contexts include mycobacterial DNA analyses (Bos et al. 2014). Other limitations on identifying the presence of tuberculosis in skeletal samples include environmental contamination of nonclinical mycobacterium in skeletal samples, and difficulties distinguishing between tubercular and nontubercular mycobacterium on a molecular level (Roberts and Buikstra 2003).

Clinical Diagnosis of Tuberculosis, Constitutional Pathology, and Disease Metaphors

Before the advent of modern diagnostics, eighteenth- and nineteenth-century physicians relied on constitutional medicine to evaluate a patient's risk of contracting a disease and to diagnose its presence in patients. Physicians' ability to assess a patient's risk of contracting tuberculosis required assessing their constitution. One's constitution was guided by a complex of factors such as physical appearance, moral inclinations, personality, and habits. Each patient was thought to have an individual constitution that guided their overall health. Doctors viewed personal health as a complex interplay of intellectual aptitude, morality, habits, seasons, and weather. Even the motions of the heavens could affect a person's health (Bivins 2013: 8). Fundamental to "constitutional pathology" was the notion that intellectual acuity, moral character, and physical health were intrinsically linked (Haller 1981). Physicians argued that individuals with so-called weak constitutions and "feeble minds" were more apt to suffer from diseases like tuberculosis, while individuals who were intelligent, hardworking, and had a strong moral foundation were less prone to experiencing disease (Haller 1981).

By acquiring knowledge of a patient's temperament, physicians were thought to be better positioned to evaluate their susceptibility to specific diseases and offer suitable courses of treatment (Haller 1981). The AMA stated in 1847 that "a medical man who has become acquainted with the peculiarities of constitution, habits, and predispositions, of those he attends, is more likely to be successful in his treatments" (Haller 1981: 18). Individuals with "sanguine constitutions" were believed to be more vulnerable to tuberculosis and other lung infections, venereal diseases, pneumonia, pleurisy, and hemorrhages. These pathologies required venesection as a primary means of treatment. "Bilious persons" were prone to diseases of the organs and were thought to be suited to mercury treatments (Haller 1981: 19). Following the development of bacteriology and immunology in medicine and their general acceptance among medical professionals, theories of constitution still continued to inform medical diagnosis, treatment, and public health policy governing tuberculosis well into the twentieth century (Haller 1981; Pagel 1955).

Even after Robert Koch identified the tuberculosis bacterium in 1882 as the cause of clinical tuberculosis, the central tenets of constitutional pathology continued to capture the social imagination of Victorian-era America and England (Dormandy 2000; Ott 1996; Pagel 1955). For the privileged middle classes, consumption was as much a physiological condition as a mental, emotional, and even spiritual state of existence. Being diagnosed with tuberculosis was a way of self-fashioning related to certain religious experiences, melancholia, physical beauty, and creative ability (Byrne 2011; Day 2017; Lawlor and Suzuki 2000; Mason et al. 2016). Writers, artists, and laypeople romanticized the symptoms of consumption; victims were often described as pale, thin, and beautiful with radiant skin and glowing eyes (Roberts 2020). In short, it was the "most flattering of all diseases" (Ott 1996: 10). "Consumption set the standard for white, middle-class beauty in the mid-nineteenth century. The image of pale, bedridden, wasting women and men quickened the pulse of Victorian readers both here and abroad" (Ott 1996: 13). The medical profession and the general public reinforced the desirable social identities attributed to tuberculosis (Byrne 2011: 12). Writers waxed poetic about the intellectual and imaginative virtues that were bestowed upon consumptives, in addition to the consumptive's physically attractive qualities (Daniel et al. 2014). These traits were reinforced in medical literature, as physicians often remarked on the "amiability" and the talents, gifts, and beauty of their consumptive patients (Byrne 2011: 20). Even though tuberculosis patients nearly always died of the disease after suffering for many years, the end stages of tuberculosis were also romanticized (Figure 4.2); women in particular were admired for their "flushed cheeks and bright eyes" during the end stages of illness (Byrne 2011). The lived realities of tuberculosis existed in stark contrast to the romanticized representations ascribed to the disease by wealthy Victorians (Bynum 2012).

Despite the prevalence of tuberculosis in the Americas since the 1700s, physicians did not consider it a public health concern until the 1840s. In Britain and France, the medical community's interest in tuberculosis did not correlate with increased incidence of the disease, but rather was coterminous with its new social significance (Byrne 2011). In contrast to tuberculosis's earlier, romantic image, by the mid-nineteenth century, the

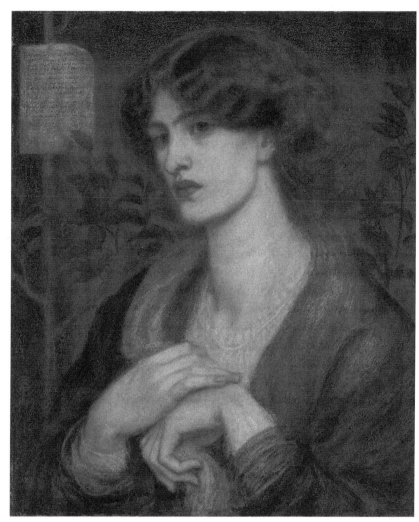

Figure 4.2. Dante Gabriel Rossetti's painting, *The Salutation of Beatrice* (1869). The artist's consumptive wife Elizabeth Siddal is portrayed as the character Beatrice from Dante Alighieri's *La Vita Nuova*. Wikimedia Commons, public domain.

disease became synonymous with its own widespread incidence among the working classes. Tuberculosis was equated with the failure of society as a whole (Bynum 2012). This signified a far departure from the idyllic, romanticized versions that permeated middle- and upper-class representations of the disease. By the 1870s and 1880s, developments in urban public health policy, bacteriology, and urban reform movements changed how specialists and the general public interpreted tuberculosis in poor, immigrant, and working-class populations.

After Koch's discovery that tuberculosis is an infectious disease caused by bacilli, physicians argued that external factors, such as climate, *caused* consumption in people who were already constitutionally *predisposed* to it (Craddock 1998: 59). Tuberculosis was thought to reside within individuals with weak constitutions, undisciplined work habits, and preexisting health conditions. In short, the consumptive possessed an "imaginary anatomy" (Craddock 1998); "it served to make a difficult-to-diagnose disease easily visible, it marked the tubercular off from the normative healthy body, and it designated a set of characteristics increasingly suspect in an industrial milieu which depended on productivity and the physical discipline of the worker" (Craddock 1998: 60). And, as Rosenberg (1977) argues, the association of disease with deviance had enormous social implications, namely by rendering disease etiologies a form of social control and a rationale for legitimating social and political inequality.

By the 1850s and 1860s, physicians and public health authorities began to interpret tuberculosis in working-class populations through interlocking lenses of race, class, gender, and citizenship status (Abel 1997, 2007; Craddock 1998). Craddock (2000) argues that by the early twentieth century, tuberculosis became a trope for civic degeneracy; as such, it provided an impetus for moral reform and nation building. Curing tuberculosis was as much about technical innovation, diagnostic techniques, and innovative medical treatment as it was about social engineering. The relationship between citizenship status and health underscores the claim by Rose and Novas (2005: 439) that "specific biological suppositions, explicitly or implicitly, have underlain many citizenship projects, shaped conceptions of what it means to be a citizen, and underpinned distinctions between actual, potential, troublesome, and impossible citizens." As the authors argue, "biocitizenship" corresponds to nationalist projects that link citizenship, political rights, and responsibilities to specific biological states. Governments and institutions manage citizens partly through biological terms of belonging (Lupton 1993: 427). Consumption, then, provided a central point for broader conversations regarding what it meant to be a good US citizen. Consumption was overwhelmingly framed by public health authorities, physicians, and reformers as a moral failing linked to the alleged laziness and "filth" of immigrant communities (Bynum 2012). Tuberculosis rhetoric mirrored eugenics discourses about the "immigrant problem"

(Craddock 2001: 344) and public perceptions that immigrant populations and associated diseases and poverty were degrading the American quality of life. The goals of anti-tuberculosis campaigns were thus twofold: to protect "native" Americans from infectious diseases located within immigrant communities and to elevate the citizenship status of poor, immigrant populations via moral reform and education programs.

Case Study: San Francisco and the Bay Area, California

San Francisco, California, had one of the largest populations of tuberculosis patients in the United States during the nineteenth century. Unsurprisingly, then, the tuberculosis landscape of San Francisco and the larger Bay Area has been well studied from historical perspectives. Large population movements in the mid-1800s, as a result of the Gold Rush and immigration, made San Franciscan citizens particularly susceptible to changing disease ecologies (Buzon et al. 2005). Despite historical statistics that suggest in the years between 1800 and 1900 over 35,000 people in San Francisco died from tuberculosis, the disease was not given considerable attention by city and county public health constituencies until the early twentieth century (Craddock 2000). The reasons for the initial lack of public health oversight are complex. For one, tuberculosis was not considered communicable during the nineteenth century (Dormandy 2000). Second, tuberculosis epidemics were seemingly erratic and spatially unfixed. Unlike cholera and smallpox, which were decidedly racialized and metonymous with San Francisco's Chinatown and poorer neighborhoods, tuberculosis infected individuals from all social classes and racial groups (Craddock 1995, 1999). Tuberculosis was seemingly nowhere and everywhere at once. Because of its spatial unfixity, individuals who were "haunted by the disease" were largely ignored by public health officials and San Francisco housing authorities until the late nineteenth century (Craddock 2000).

Following the Civil War, public health discourses in the United States increasingly instilled tuberculosis's associations with poverty and unsanitary living conditions. As Craddock (2000: 65) notes, the "slum body" served as a potent metaphor for the degraded urban landscape. Changes in public health mapping technologies, especially the development of spot maps in the early 1900s, meant that public health authorities and physicians could visually "prove" that high tuberculosis rates coincided with poorer, immigrant neighborhoods. By 1869, the ontology of tuberculosis became synonymous with the city's underclass neighborhoods and slums. By 1870, it became clear from California State Board of Health records that rising tuberculosis rates no longer resulted from external migration, but represented an endemic crisis born of crowding, "immoral slums," and "degraded structural surroundings" (Craddock 1998: 65). The poor, particularly immigrants, were explicitly blamed by public health authorities and physicians for perpetuating the conditions and spread of "their" disease. Tuberculosis was increasingly spatialized; infected city spaces became coterminous with the infected bodies that inhabited them (Craddock 1998, 2000). In reality, San Francisco's unprecedented tuberculosis rates were likely precipitated by crowded neighborhoods, overburdened hospitals and poorhouses, and administrative failures by local government to facilitate adequate living and working conditions (Craddock 2000: 43). Crowding in San Francisco's SOMA neighborhood became chronic and severe during the 1870s and 1880s, which facilitated the spread of the disease.

Statistical studies illuminated the vast discrepancies in tuberculosis rates between working- and middle-class urban neighborhoods. Progressive Era reformers rallied to improve housing and sewer systems in poorer San Francisco neighborhoods (Craddock 1998), while the reordering of social life (Soja 1996) hastened wealthier residents' moves to outlying areas of the city such as North Beach and the Presidio. Treatments for tuberculosis also had a distinctly geographic quality. Wealthy "consumptives" and "tuberculars" flocked to cities across the United States that claimed to have a salubrious and healthy climate, perfect for healing afflicted lungs. Upper- and middle-class consumptives traveled to elite sanatoria in New York, Southern California, and Colorado (Abel 2007). During the 1850s and 1860s, San Francisco ironically became a principal area of respite for local and migrant tuberculosis patients (Craddock 2000) and, paradoxically, physicians and public health authorities welcomed wealthy tubercular migrants into San Francisco.

Beginning in the early twentieth century, public health measures were initiated to protect wealthier neighborhoods from working-class tuberculars (Craddock 2000). These measures included placing tuberculosis patients in county and city hospitals, whether voluntarily or forcibly, and removing working-class tuberculars from the city in order to place them in rural tuberculosis sanatoria. Public health authorities and city planners argued that removing working-class patients from the city reduced the threat of disease to middle- and upper-class neighborhoods as "poor and infected bodies advanced inexorably across urban topographies" (Craddock 2000: 163). Working-class sanatoria in the early twentieth century were designed to contain patients within an open-air environment and offer them medical treatments in exchange for pay or labor. Importantly, sanatoria activities were designed to "produce vigorous, strong bodies from weak ones" through a strict regimen of exercise and job training programs (Craddock 2000). The twin goals of institutionally supported work programs were to keep working-class individuals accustomed to the type of work routine to which they would inevitably return, while also "staving off the proclivities of idleness presumed characteristic of the urban poor" (Craddock 2000: 174).

Archaeological and historical research on twentieth-century tuberculosis sanatoria in Northern California illustrates how etiologies and curative methods reinforced normative ideas about the body, respectable behavior, and well-being (Scott 2023). Specifically, Scott focuses on consumptive spaces, demonstrating how the built environment of sanatoria was meant to show how tuberculosis could be controlled through certain practices such as rest, sunbathing, and consuming specific foods (Scott 2023: 205). Scott specifically highlights window glass recovered from sanatoria in Placer County and Colfax, California, to examine how glass functioned as a medical technology in these spaces and embodied specific social expectations regarding behavior, bodies, race, gender, and normative abilities. She examines how normative discourses regarding health and ableism affected practices, the body, and the built environment within California sanatoria. She furthermore uses medical and social models of disability to examine how these models normatively shaped definitions of tuberculosis, its treatment, and perceptions of patients' bodies and behavior. She argues that the "normative body which was aspired to at TB sanatoria was a body which was free from tuberculosis" (Scott 2023: 205). This was accomplished through rest, access to sunlight, and diet. Scott interprets the window glass at Weimar Joint Sanatorium and Colfax Sanatorium as a form of medical technology, insofar as it allowed beneficial sunlight and air to reach patients. This spatial environment of fresh air and sunlight facilitated lifestyle changes in patients and was meant to shape tubercular bodies into healthy ones.

Another well-studied institution in California is Arequipa Sanatorium. In 1911, San Francisco physician Philip King Brown (1914, 1919) constructed the Arequipa Sanatorium for Working Women in Marin County. Brown established Arequipa specifically for working-class women, with the aim of removing them from harmful factory work and teaching them middle-class values, including domesticity and home health (Brown 1914; Downey 1994). Since tuberculosis symbolized the social, moral, and economic failings of working-class society, treatment necessitated ridding bodies of the disease through the reproduction of middle-class values, especially in women (Craddock 2001). As keepers of the home and family, women were seen as the primary means through which personal and family health could be achieved. While medicine at large was increasingly institutionalized during the late nineteenth and early twentieth centuries, "the home" became the primary locus of tuberculosis prevention and treatment. Tuberculosis sanatoria adopted domestic "attitudes" and sought to present as "homelike" to their patients (Craddock 2001: 340). Rhetorical strategies used by physicians and reformers exhibited eugenic overtones; women were responsible not only for maintaining the health of their families but also for securing the health of the nation. Immigration was framed as a direct threat to the well-being of the United States, and (white) middle-class women were key players in medical campaigns that promoted the production of (white) children and the maintenance of family health (Craddock 2001: 344). As Craddock (2001) notes, eugenics discourses and policies did not focus solely on sexual reproduction; the poor and immigrant classes could be brought into the "fold of civilization" through behavior modification and living improvements.

At Arequipa Sanatorium, Brown held conventional beliefs concerning the relationship between unhealthy environments and the spread of tuberculosis, viewing the cramped, close quarters of working-class women as a fundamental factor. One of Brown's goals was to remove working-class women from deleterious working and living conditions and place them in healthful environments. In many ways, Brown's concern for the well-being of working-class women was historically unprecedented; few treatment facilities catered specifically to women (Downey 2019). Despite Brown's novel concern for working-class women, his theories regarding treatment generally aligned with public eugenics theories of the time (Craddock 2001: 346). Brown only accepted young, white women. He specified that only the "intelligent, teachable type [of woman] is selected for admittance, and only those allowed to remain who prove amenable to discipline. This policy results in a student body . . . which becomes in time . . . a real force in public health education" (Brown 1911). Brown's statement suggests that women contracted consumption in part through their moral failings and that they could be healed through the reproduction of middle-class values (Craddock 2001).

At the sanatorium, women were subject to a range of regulations. They could not eat or sleep outside of normal hours, nor could they leave the grounds without permission or visit other patients (Craddock 2000: 183). For patients at Arequipa, only work understood as suitable for females was permitted. Women were assigned occupations that appealed to the "feminine instincts of personal adornment and homebuilding" and provided them with vocational skills that might serve them upon leaving the institution (Craddock 2000). Women grew their own food, participated in light construction activities, and produced crafts for sale to help fund their treatment (Downey 1994, 2019). Many patients at Arequipa also made pottery as part of their training and healing process (Downey 2019; Harley and Schwartz 2013). Arequipa potters were trained in the arts and crafts tradition, and pottery making was seen as both a means of paying for the costs of the stay and a therapeutic craft (Harley and Schwartz 2013). Today, Arequipa pottery is highly sought after as a collector's item.

Women who were "cured" of tuberculosis (meaning those whose symptoms subsided) were allowed to leave the sanatorium and return to a more "enlightened" and healthy life in the city. As Craddock notes, the irony was that the middle-class, feminine training programs at Arequipa did not resemble the industrial settings to which most Arequipa patients would return (Craddock 2000: 184). Furthermore, women rarely left sanatoria and state hospitals permanently once their symptoms subsided. Most patients opted for care at home but were forced to return frequently to hospitals and sanitaria to receive what they and their families perceived to be adequate care.

In 1957, the sanatorium at Arequipa closed, and the buildings were torn down in 1984 (Downey 1994). In 1989, the camp and surrounding property were permanently donated to the Girl Scouts of the San Francisco Bay Area. The Arequipa Girl Scout Camp mission statement pays homage to the history of the sanatorium by stating, somewhat ironically (in *The Independent Journal's* editorial of November 8, 1961), "What more fitting thing could be done with it [Arequipa] than to rededicate it to our future, the women of tomorrow? What better use for it than to train the girls to be better women and citizens of tomorrow?" (Camp Arequipa 2024).

Bottom-Up Perspectives on Tuberculosis

Histories of medicine have recently adopted bottom-up approaches that foreground the experiences of patients, and in doing so, deviate from policy- and doctor-centered narratives. By analyzing firsthand accounts of tuberculosis patients, including diaries and correspondences, social historians have been able to understand the relationship between subjective experiences of disease and macrosocial and political structures (Bates 1992). Scholars have also adopted critical approaches to contemporary anti-tuberculosis programs by situating them within their social and historical contexts. An example includes Farmer's (2000) critique of the concept of "noncompliance." He argues that patients' inability to complete tuberculosis treatments and participate in targeted initiatives is not due to personal ambivalence but rather is rooted in social conditions that make participation difficult, if not impossible (Farmer 2000).

Although archaeological research on tuberculosis institutions is less common than work focusing on other public health organizations (such as asylums and public hospitals), archaeological research can provide an important window into the subjective experience of living with tuberculosis. This work provides an intimate understanding of how individuals and communities coped with tuberculosis and how they negotiated targeted public health policies. As Rose and Novas (2005) argue, biocitizenship is not only imposed "from above" by governments and regulatory agencies, but these projects also shape subjective understandings of self. How do normative biomedical classifications affect citizen groups who are targeted by health discourses and policies? How do public health discourses and practical measures shape citizens' understandings of self? How do they impact material practices associated with self-care?

Archaeological studies have addressed these questions within the broader historical and social contexts in which individuals with tuberculosis navigated institutionalized racism, classism, and prohibitive access to professional care. For example, Linn's (2008) archaeological and archival analyses of health conditions among Irish Americans in nineteenth-century New York demonstrate that tuberculosis was a harrowing, lived reality for immigrant communities. Hospital and dispensary records indicate that Irish Americans suffered from the highest rates of tuberculosis due to crowded living conditions, insufficient diet, and occupations like masonry and carpentry that precipitated respiratory infections (Linn 2008: 469). Physicians and public health authorities viewed tuberculosis as "naturalized" among immigrant populations in New York and thus left care for the disease largely to the patients (Linn 2008: 447). Artifacts and macrobotanical remains recovered from Five Points and Patterson, New York, suggest that Irish families used a range of healing practices to abate symptoms of tuberculosis, including medicinal plants, foods, and patent medicines. Macrobotanical analyses indicate that Irish American families may have used blackberry, cherry, dock, elderberry, mint, and sorrel plants to aid in treating symptoms. Patent medicine bottles from products advertised as blood purifiers, cough remedies, and painkillers were also recovered from the two contexts (Linn 2008: 509). These patent medicines would have been widely available and would have also helped to counter the symptoms of tuberculosis. Archaeological case studies such as Linn's provide a bottom-up perspective, showing how communities most at risk for tuberculosis navigated disease symptoms and the broader political milieus that framed them, such as prohibitive access to care and anti-immigrant policies.

Conclusion

As archaeologists have argued, by understanding the disasters of the past, we can anticipate effects and focus on resilience in the present, or what Riede (2017) calls "past-forwarding." By focusing on the *longue durée,* archaeologists are well positioned to investigate biological and social re-sponses to infectious disease in the past and elucidate the interconnections between past epidemics and the injustices that face marginalized commu-nities in the present (Gamble et al. 2021: 15). As DeWitte (2016: 64) notes, fundamental questions in public health concern who is most at risk of dis-ease; how social, economic, and environmental factors shape epidemics; and how epidemic diseases affect the health status of human populations over the short and long term. She further argues that contemporary poli-cymakers and health practitioners lack the temporal depth necessary to fully examine, and anticipate, the behavior of emerging diseases (DeWitte 2016).

In particular, biocultural approaches provide invaluable tools for evaluating how epidemics act on human populations, and how certain biological indicators such as age, gender, and health status impact health outcomes over the *longue durée* (Zuckerman et al. 2022). Archaeological investigation into past infectious diseases can deepen research's temporal scope regarding their causes and consequences, thus providing better tools for mitigating disease in contemporary living populations. Long-term per-spectives help to identify vulnerable populations and predict which fac-tors are most likely to lead to negative health outcomes (DeWitte 2016: 71). Archaeological inquiries, which are temporally sensitive, can also demon-strate how pandemics are not intermittent disasters—infectious diseases have long lifespans and thus have extended temporalities and broad geo-graphic scales. Epidemics are also not isolated, biological events, but are rather embedded in sociopolitical processes. As public health responses to COVID-19 illustrated, social inequalities (for example, lack of access to healthcare, income inequality, racism, etc.) exacerbate pandemics, and further entrench unequal social relations. Archaeologists are equipped to move beyond disease modeling to illustrate the social transformations that shaped and were shaped by disease responses.

Also, medicine and public health do not operate independently of social politics; rather, politics are embedded within the very structures of public health. Power is implicated in the ways that "vulnerability" and "suscepti-bility" are framed in public health discourse (Lupton 1993). As the studies in this chapter demonstrate, scholars must be aware of how they frame vulnerability and risk in their research. The archaeological examples here demonstrate how the identification of "vulnerable" and "at risk" biological beings has been intrinsically linked to normative standards of morality, compliance, and good citizenship. Public health policy developed not as a means to secure the health statuses of entire populations, but as a way to protect those who were deemed worthy of health and identify those in need of structural reform. Structural inequalities are built into the public healthcare system and archaeologists are in a unique position to study the historical trajectories of healthcare inequalities, examine the experience of infectious disease in the past, and inform public health perspectives in the present.

5

Biocitizenship and Healthcare at the Presidio of San Francisco

The Moral Imperative of Health and Hygiene

Citizenship has an enduring relationship with the human body. The associations between the body, public health, and citizenship are demonstrated by nineteenth- and twentieth-century policies regarding eugenics, women's reproductive rights, and domestic health campaigns targeting immigrant populations (Happe et al. 2018). This set of relations between bodies, political regulation, and citizenship has recently become known as "biocitizenship." Theories of biocitizenship, drawing from Foucauldian theories of biopolitics that stress the state's disciplinary power over the body, claim that the physical body and its health are fundamental to the citizen subject (Johnson et al. 2018). Biocitizenship is also a generative concept, since it outlines the necessary conditions required for political action and participation within the state (Johnson et al. 2018). Thus, biocitizenship reforms bodies, but also provides certain rights in social and political life. This chapter draws on previous discussions of public health and mobilizes the idea of biocitizenship as a guiding concept to explore how during the late nineteenth and early twentieth centuries, the US Army managed the health of enlisted soldiers to develop effectual fighters, but also to create a new generation of American citizens.

During the first half of the twentieth century, the US Army War Department aimed to shape a more efficient type of soldier, and by extension, a superior American citizen (Bristow 1996). "Military citizenship" was defined in accordance with specific prescriptive policies concerning physical health, fitness, and moral character. US Army War Department policies were influenced by broader national discourses concerning biological identification and standard ideals of hygiene, sexuality, and morality (Bristow 1996). These ideals provided a framework for specific standards of hygiene and health to which US citizens were expected to conform. Progressive Era discourses concerning "social hygiene" (a euphemism for sexual health and sexual practices) were co-opted by US Army administrations, who likewise promoted soldiers' sexual purity and abstinence from drugs, alcohol, and other "immoral" behaviors (Bristow 1996). The US War Department argued that a pure corpus and moral aptitudes not only contributed to soldiers' ability to fight in times of conflict, but also shaped them into ideal American citizens in postwar periods.

This chapter focuses on enlisted soldiers' healthcare and hygiene practices at the Presidio of San Francisco. Building rehabilitation projects from 2008–2009 at the Presidio's Montgomery Street Barracks recovered items that had been left in the barracks by enlisted soldiers, mainly from the soffit boxes (or eaves) of the buildings. Objects include military manuals, clothing items, food detritus, letters and postcards, and items such as alcohol bottles, cigarette packaging, and medications. The eaves provided convenient places for disposing of mundane objects, although some of the items may have been purposefully hidden to avoid detection during room inspections. This chapter focuses on artifacts that were used in personal care, such as patent and OTC medicines, hygiene products, and recreational drugs. I use these items to examine the relationship between Army standards of hygiene and healthcare and enlisted men's self-care practices. In addition to the archaeological evidence, this chapter presents historical and archival data on healthcare in the form of written medical texts and pamphlets as well as historical documents concerning twentieth-century healthcare and hygiene regulations in the Army.

The incredible preservation and uniqueness of these materials provide an opportunity to examine the everyday lives of enlisted soldiers during the first half of the twentieth century. They also allow an examination of the complex relationships between healthcare reform movements, military regulation, and individual healthcare routines during the early twentieth century. In this chapter, I demonstrate how self-care practices reference broader discourses concerning citizenship. While many of the objects found at the Presidio suggest that soldiers engaged with healthcare standards developed by the Army Medical Department, it is also evident that soldiers did so in ways that made sense to them. The specific brands of healthcare items found, in addition to the presence of substances banned by the military, suggest that self-care was shaped by micro-scale and macro-scale processes. Sexual responsibility, bodily hygiene, and abstinence from drugs and alcohol were the terms of military belonging and good citizenship, yet in practice, soldiers often interpreted these ideals in ways that were not envisioned by the US Army Medical Department.

This study of personal care practices at the Presidio contributes to a growing body of research in archaeology that focuses on the power dynamics between public health policies and patients' negotiation of prescriptive measures. Similar themes in archaeological studies include how individuals and households responded to sanitation, preventative medicine, and the professionalization of the healthcare sector (Fisher et al. 2007; Heffner 2015; Linn 2010). Relatedly, there has also been a surge of anthropological research on the intersection between self-care and moral and political economies (de Klerk and Moyer 2017; Lamb 2019; Montesi 2020). In anthropology, care remains a shifting concept, "alternately referring to everyday practices, engagements with biomedicine, biopolitics, affective states, forms of moral experience and obligation, structures of exploitation, and the relationships between these various things" (Buch 2015: 279). As both archaeologists and anthropologists have shown, "self-care" provides an important fulcrum point for studying the intersections between healthcare policy, social politics, and the citizen-self. Analysis of artifacts from the Presidio barracks indicates that soldiers performed self-care practices that were mandated by the US Army, but also used alternative therapies for self-care. Rather than framing self-care and alternative medicine as a rejection of conventional medicine, I argue that all care practices (including alternative medicines) represent taking a personal responsibility for health that references specific moral attitudes.

Citizenship, Biocitizenship, and Belonging

Citizenship includes status (membership and access), rights that are connected to that status, and identity that is articulated in relation to a specific political collectivity (Joppke 2007). A political collectivity may be a state, government agency, or polity. In this case study, I use *citizenship* to refer to the rights and responsibilities of enlisted soldiers as imparted by the US Army. I also use *citizenship* in its broader sense to refer to the rights and responsibilities of citizen subjects in the United States.

As for *biocitizenship*, scholars have used the term to explain how citizenship rights and responsibilities become connected to biological states of being and biosocial identities (Greenhough 2014; Johnson et al. 2018; Petryna 2004; Rose and Novas 2005). In her study of post-Chernobyl Ukraine, Petryna (2004) shows how Ukrainian citizens who were exposed to radiation argued for rights to health services and social support from the government as a result of their distinct health conditions. This study demonstrates how a large segment of Ukraine's population negotiated social, economic, and political inclusion in biological terms (Petryna 2004). Rose and Novas's (2005) definition of *biocitizenship* includes the ways that collectivities mobilize specific medical technologies as forms of self-identification. They argue that biological citizenship is both anatomizing and collectivizing. It is individualizing in the sense that self-description and self-judgment are entangled with one's "regime of the self" (Rose and Novas 2005: 134), but biological citizenship is also collectivizing in that groups of individuals galvanize "biosocialities" around a shared biological identity. These biological identities may include certain identities constructed around chronic diseases, physical aptitudes or strengths, or ideas concerning one's biological state of vulnerability and risk (Rabinow 2005).

Other definitions of *biocitizenship* more narrowly focus on moral biocitizenship (Lupton 1993). This concept describes the way that groups with similar bodily outlooks stress the importance of personal responsibility for maintaining physical health. For example, researchers who study obesity and weight loss have noted how individuals who exhibit mindful control over their bodies index themselves as moral biocitizens and aspirationally healthy individuals (SturtzSreetharan et al. 2018: 222). Examinations of moral biocitizenship foreground how "risk" may be framed by individuals and institutions as a consequence of personal lifestyle choices. In this sense of the term, the goals of health policies are to promote awareness of the dangers of certain lifestyle choices and encourage individuals to participate in health promotion and education programs (Lupton 1993: 427).

The specific case studies in this chapter are understood in relation to the last iteration of biocitizenship as moral duty and responsibility in response to health promotion campaigns. Biological citizenship includes strategies imposed by organizational structures and agencies, but also incorporates the ways in which individuals understand their rights, nationality, and terms of belonging in biological terms (Lupton 1993; Rose and Novas 2005). "Moral biocitizenship" was territorialized by the US Army along both military and civilian lines. The US Army Medical Department developed strict regulations concerning what enlisted soldiers were allowed to do with their bodies. Mandates included physical exercise and healthy eating, abstaining from sex, alcohol, and other drugs, and even refraining from using patent and OTC medications. Part of the US Army's concern was to protect the physical fitness and fighting capacity of soldiers in times of conflict. But changing discourses before and during World War II increasingly viewed soldiers as valuable "potential" citizens; by shaping the moral character of its soldiers, the Army could subsequently elevate the moral standing of soldiers-cum-citizens during postwar periods (Bristow 1996). Thus, the Army saw the soldiers' character and health status as a microcosm of American citizenry writ large.

American Citizenship and the US Army

American citizenship during the nineteenth century was "contractual, volitional, and legal rather than natural and immutable" (Hosek et al. 2020: 2). As Hosek and colleagues (2020) note, American political institutions mobilized notions of moral "character" as a rallying point around which to model citizenship. Cleanliness, health, and diet were integral to democratic citizenship. During the nineteenth and early twentieth centuries, hygiene and proper self-care were essential to practices of national belonging. Social reformers specifically targeted immigrant communities, economically disadvantaged households, and laborers who they thought were capable of self-determination and participation in civic life—but only once they conformed to middle-class values concerning health and hygiene (Linn 2008).

At the turn of the twentieth century, discursive strategies linked military participation with good citizenship. Being a "good" citizen meant participating in a normative culture of volunteerism, particularly in respect to the expanding American industrial-military complex (Capozzola 2008). The militarization of American culture and forcible military participation came to a head in 1917, when President Wilson authorized the Selective Service Act, which required citizens to register for military service (Capozzola 2008: 21). This act legitimized wartime citizenship by blurring the boundaries between political and military obligations and framing national belonging in terms of military support. During both World Wars, the US military claimed to have distributed the civic duty to protect the country across all male US citizens (Amaya 2007: 4).

Despite nationalistic discourses and policies that framed military participation as equally distributed among American men, US military recruitment practices historically targeted poor and immigrant communities (Amaya 2007). During the Spanish-American War and the World Wars, recruitment practices targeted recent immigrants, members of rural communities, and other members of economically marginalized social groups (Coffman 2009). During World War I, the US government drafted into service almost half a million immigrants. This created a large army of soldiers who were born overseas (Ford 2011: 3). For recent immigrants and economically disadvantaged men, joining the Army as an enlisted soldier was a way to elevate one's social and economic position. For members of the regular or standing Army, enlistment was often a last resort for those who had other prospects for securing the steady income that was "essential to family formation and citizenship" (Guardino 2014: 26). Enlistment came with a number of demanding responsibilities and duties, but it also came with rights and security in terms of a paid career, economic support, and access to educational programs (Coffman 2009).

During the end of the nineteenth century and first half of the twentieth century, military institutions like the Army worked closely with Progressive reformers to develop programs that would help to "Americanize" enlisted soldiers (Ford 2011). In 1917, the War Department hired prominent Progressive Era social reformers to consult on military moral uplift and "Americanization" strategies. These hires included Raymond Fosdick, John Mott (secretary of the Young Men's Christian Association of America [YMCA]), and Secretary of War Newton Baker, a municipal Progressive reformer (Ford 2011: 9). The goals of social welfare organizations like the YMCA and Knights of Columbus in the US military were to socialize and shape the moral character of native-born and foreign-born soldiers alike (Petit 2021). At the Presidio of San Francisco, the Army enlisted the help of the Knights of Columbus and the YMCA to provide for the needs of Catholic and Christian soldiers (Thompson 1997). These organizations promoted social welfare programs that were meant to keep soldiers away from the negative influences of prostitution, gambling, and alcohol by providing wholesome alternatives (Slominski 2021).

Citizenship and Moral Character Programs

After the Spanish-American War in 1898, the War Department and civilian societies voiced concerns regarding alcohol, transmissible disease, and sex among US servicemen in Cuba, the Philippines, and Puerto Rico (Cirillo 2004). By World War I, the US government was undertaking a sweeping effort to suppress "vice" among servicemen overseas and at home by remaking their moral character. This included protecting them from self-medication, alcohol, sex, and other "untoward" behaviors (Reilly 2014: 225). The War Department also took an opportunity to shape the moral character of soldiers who would become citizens at the end of the war. Once soldiers' moral character was linked to national identity, "the moral failures of America's fighting force would stand as a measure of the unfitness of the citizenry" (Reilly 2014: 225). While European militaries also developed policies to curb alcohol consumption, drug use, and sex among their own servicemen, the United States was touted as "the most aggressively moral nation on earth" (Reilly 2014: 226).

US military policies regarding soldiers' health were not merely a materialization of concerns regarding physical fitness, nor were they an extension of Progressive Era reform movements (Reilly 2014). Rather, they encapsulated broader debates concerning American imperialism, national belonging, and civic identity. American discourses around questions of citizenship revealed the anxieties of US officials and the public over the racial, ethnic, and class identities of enlisted soldiers and their ultimate capacity for citizenship and self-governance (Bristow 1996). The War Department's programs aimed to provide recruits with wholesome activities such as athletics, motion pictures, and chaperoned parties. Army education programs, such as the Commission on Training Camp Activities (CTCA), were an attempt to instill white, middle-class values in servicemen and functionally erase class, ethnic, racial, and religious differences within military and civilian society (Reilly 2014: 227). The War Department developed the CTCA in 1917 to "prevent inefficiency in fighting forces endangered by drunkenness and disease . . . by civilian moral uplifting work" (Ford 2011: 88). The War Department hoped that recreational and educational programs would forge an "invisible armor" (Reilly 2014: 235) of moral social habits and improve soldiers' moral purity and biological well-being. This retraining would forge a new kind of biocitizen, one who would overcome his biological and racial "shortcomings" to become a productive, assimilated member of civilian society. At the Presidio, several wholesome recreational activities were available. Although one soldier noted that the Presidio was "the most liberally controlled Army post in the United States," it also offered "rides through the hills and hikes along the beaches[;] if the soldier desired indoor recreation . . . there were the YMCA buildings and the Red Cross Club Room in the Oregon Building" (Ford 2011).

Venereal diseases were of particular concern to the Army since they were thought to negatively reflect on a soldier's moral character (Figure 5.1). In 1917, the Social Hygiene Division of the Commission on Training Camp Activities was established, based on a curriculum developed by the Army Surgeon General. The official pamphlet, entitled *Keeping Fit to Fight,* was introduced to all enlisted men in training camps (Bristow 1996: 34). The pamphlet was meant to serve two purposes: to provide sexual health education to enlisted soldiers, and to warn soldiers that if they contracted

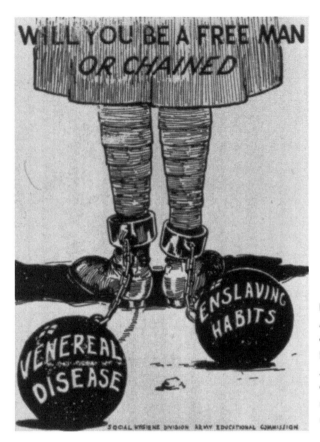

Figure 5.1. *Will You Be a Free Man or Chained?* Social Hygiene Division, Army Educational Commission. Wikimedia Commons, public domain.

venereal disease, it would be a disgrace to both their families and the US government. The pamphlet was translated for soldiers whose reading language was not English (Ford 2011). Similarly, the film version of *Keeping Fit to Fight* was translated into foreign languages in the hope that the message would reach foreign-born troops (Ford 2011: 101). The pamphlet stated that any form of self-treatment or the use of "quack medicines" for venereal disease would not be tolerated (American Social Hygiene Association 1918: 9). Relatedly, the Army General Order No. 17 of 1912 required soldiers who may have been exposed to venereal disease to seek treatment from Army doctors within a matter of hours after exposure (Allen 1918). Failure to seek and follow recommended treatment would spur trial by court-martial and being relieved of duty (Allen 1918: 169). All soldiers who exposed themselves to venereal disease would incur a stoppage of pay and restriction of privileges while under treatment (Allen 1918: 169).

The Army's concern for the sexual health of soldiers could be traced to the soldiers' camps along the US-Mexico border during the Spanish-American War. A quote from the Army's 1898 medical regulations describes the dangers of sexual liaisons: "When a young man is 'sowing his wild oats' he is really planting in his own body the syphilis and clap plants, and the harvest will be greater than any other crop. He will reap it in days of bed-ridden misery, and possible sudden death. He will reap it in bitter hours by the bedside through the illness and death of his wife or in her long years of ill health . . . Yes, the wild oats is a bumper crop" (Allen 1918: 171). Recognizing that soldiers would inevitably engage in sex, the Army Medical Department also developed strict protocols for dealing with sexually transmitted infections. The 1898 medical regulations state, "Should you discover that you have clap or other venereal disease, report to the hospital at once for treatment. You will receive the best possible treatment and it will cost you nothing. Don't commit the error of attempting to hide your misfortune or of going to some cheap civilian doctor in hopes of keeping the facts from the military authorities" (Allen 1918: 172). Syphilis treatments, in the form of a "K-pack," could be purchased from post exchanges or acquired from post physicians (Bristow 1996).

Alcohol use in the military was similarly a rallying point for social welfare campaigns. During the Prohibition movement, soldiers' alcohol use was criticized by the Women's Christian Temperance Union (WCTU) and members of Congress (Bristow 1996). These critics pushed for the abolition of alcohol in American society, in both civilian and military establishments. The political debate over alcohol sales, consumption, and the US Army mirrored broader societal concerns regarding individual consent, freedom of choice, and government regulation (Baker 2016). The canteen and alcohol debate also revealed the American public's complicated opinions about soldiers and generated concern regarding the moral and social conditions of the Army (Baker 2016: 723). Paternalist and maternalist discourses regarding soldiers' welfare and health were prevalent among social reformers; soldiers were often described in protective terms, as "boys" in need of help and guidance (Baker 2016: 720). Policies in the Army against drinking overwhelmingly targeted the working classes and ethnic minorities (Wintermute 2010). In 1891, the Surgeon General's office reported that enlisted soldiers of Irish descent had the highest rate of drunkenness of any enlisted ethnic group (Wintermute 2010: 190). Similarly, German soldiers during the same time period received a disproportionate number of Army officer complaints for excessive alcohol use (Wintermute 2010).

In addition to alcohol use and social hygiene, personal hygiene also proved a fulcrum point for broader discussions concerning soldiers' health and fitness and, in turn, the aptitudes of American citizens. As Brown (2009) notes, bodily care changed drastically since the sixteenth century. Cleanliness, including personal hygiene, involves a complex regimen of private practices that reference broader public convictions regarding gender, civic duty, and labor (Brown 2009). What Brown (2009) terms "body work" included strategies for cleaning the body and keeping one's living spaces free of dirt. Seemingly mundane tasks, such as bathing, toothbrushing, douching, trimming one's nails, and hair grooming referenced broader social expectations regarding civility and simultaneously expressed broader societal fears regarding pollution and contamination. European colonialism marked the beginning of a profound shift in how Europeans (and later Americans) interpreted and performed cleanliness, which became an important marker of the line between "self" and "other" (Brown 2009). Scholars have convincingly argued that hygiene practices generally fell under the purview of women, since women were viewed as caretakers of the home and family, especially beginning in the late twentieth century. But the US military also played a significant role in shaping men's practices and expectations regarding cleanliness.

Hygiene has long been used as a method of assessment for the suitability of nonwhite populations and/or immigrants for citizenship (Horton and Barker 2009: 1). Social histories of medicine have demonstrated the extent to which personal hygiene was deemed central to public health policies on race and citizenship. Immigration to the United States between 1890 and 1920 facilitated discourses concerning the relationship between eugenics and citizenship; public health agencies were established to mediate the perceived hygienic threats that immigrant groups posed to US-born citizens. At San Francisco's Angel Island, Chinese, South Indian, and Filipino immigrants were screened for preexisting medical conditions that were thought to negatively affect their productivity as laborers, or else threatened to infect US-born citizens (Shah 2001: 86). Similarly, medical inspection plants along the US-Mexico border screened Mexican immigrants for typhus and other infectious diseases, which lent credibility to immigration policies based on eugenic standards of physical fitness.

In the US Army, discourses on hygiene were similarly embedded in middle-class (white) theories concerning morality, self-discipline, and bioracial superiority. Enlistee training camps, Army posts, and garrisons were viewed by ministers, public health officials, and military officers as hotbeds of corruption and filth. Training camps, in particular, were characterized as comprising a "heterogeneous mob" of soldiers, a "welter of dissimilar, divergent, and dangerous units of humanity" (Reilly 2014: 237). Disciplinary hygiene tactics in military establishments targeted not only immigrants, to include "Chinese laundrymen" and "Irish gangsters," but also poor, rural whites who needed to be brought into the fold of civilization (Reilly 2014: 239). Following the Civil War, the US Army increasingly shifted responsibility for daily health from the institution to the individual. Germ theories of disease, the development of sanitation technologies by the Army, such as disinfection, and broader civic concerns with respectability precipitated new, prescribed techniques of the self (Marshall 1997). The Army Medical Department prescribed quotidian hygiene measures, including keeping one's laundry and room clean, cleaning one's clothes and shoes, bathing daily with soap, and keeping nails and hair trimmed to an adequate length. Army officers frequently staged surprise inspections in which enlisted men were required to "strip to their underwear to demonstrate their cleanliness" (Coffman 2009: 103). The War Department hoped that these class-based hygiene and self-care habits would be incorporated into soldiers' home communities once their service had ended.

Biocitizenship and Self-Care at the Presidio of San Francisco

The Presidio of San Francisco provides a unique opportunity to examine how enlisted soldiers mobilized the Army's concerns with moral ascriptions of health and hygiene. The Presidio provides a useful case study through which to examine US Army discourses concerning biocitizenship and self-care through material practices. Objects found at the Presidio enlisted soldiers' barracks provide a unique opportunity to examine how self-care practices reference broader discourses concerning citizenship. The guiding frameworks and findings of this study also connect with the larger themes of this book concerning public health, consumerism and self-care, and power and inequality in medicine.

Presidio Background

In 1774, the Spanish viceroy, Antonio María Bucareli, ordered Captain Juan Bautista de Anza Bezerra Nieto to lead an expedition from Tubac, Mexico to open a route to Monterey, California (Tutorow 1996: 154). In 1776, Bucareli sent Anza on a second mission to what is now San Francisco. The Presidio of San Francisco was formally established as a military post in

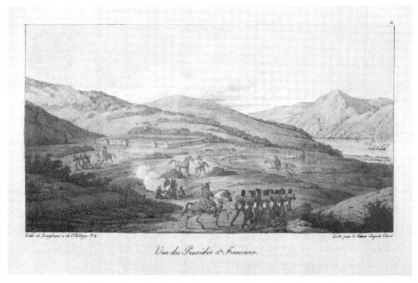

Figure 5.2. Victor Adam after Louis Choris, *Vue du Presidio san Francisco* (1822). Wikimedia Commons, public domain.

September of that year (Figure 5.2). Soldier settlers constructed an adobe fort near the Native Yelamu Ohlone village of Petlenuc (Jones 2019: 184). The Mission San Francisco de Asís was also constructed in what is now the city of San Francisco. The goal of the Spanish colonial project was to convert Native Californians to Christianity and turn them into subjects of the Spanish Crown (Blind et al. 2004). The Presidio remained under Spanish control until Mexico claimed its independence in 1822 (Tutorow 1996: 155). By 1835, the Presidio was mostly abandoned by soldiers who settled large tracts of land in Miwok and Ohlone territories (Jones 2019: 184). US military forces took control of the fort in 1846, after which the Presidio operated as a US Army post until it was decommissioned in 1994 (Thompson 1997). Today the Presidio of San Francisco is a nearly 1,500-acre park within Golden Gate National Recreation Area (Jones 2019). The park is managed by the Presidio Trust, which was created to rehabilitate and reanimate the Army post (Jones 2019: 183). The National Historic Landmark District at the Presidio includes over 400 contributing buildings, 30 archaeological areas, and cultural landscapes (Jones 2019: 184). In 2013, the trust developed the Presidio Heritage Program, which includes a heritage museum, the Archaeology Lab, and an ongoing public archaeology program (Jones 2019: 185).

The US Army took control of the Presidio in 1846, the year in which the US Army forced the transfer of California from Mexico to the United States (Thompson 1997). Over the next 148 years, the Army transformed the Presidio grounds from a Spanish fort into an important military post (Thompson 1997). US Army development projects included building hospitals, nursing units, garrisons, soldiers' barracks and commissioned officers' houses, and artillery units. In 1898, the United States declared war on Spain; the Presidio served as a post to assemble troops before deploying to the Philippines (Sokolov and Bertland 2020: 89). That same year, the Army's Surgeon General approved the construction of a General Hospital to treat sick and injured soldiers returning from the Philippines (Sokolov and Bertland 2020: 89), who suffered from typhoid fever, mumps and measles, lung diseases such as pneumonia and bronchitis, and venereal diseases. After the San Francisco earthquake and fire of 1906, the hospital also took in and cared for injured civilians (Thompson 1997). In 1911, the War Department renamed General Hospital the Letterman Hospital, after Major Jonathan Letterman (Sokolov and Bertland 2020). Aside from Walter Reed Hospital in Washington, DC, the Letterman Hospital was the only US Army General Hospital operating at the beginning of the twentieth century.

After the Army's acquisition of the Presidio in 1846, Colonel Mansfield expressed concern over the poor quality of the soldiers' living accommodations: "The quarters for the soldiers were miserable adobe buildings, the leavings of the Mexican government . . . a temporary barrack for the soldiers has been subsequently erected by order of the General [John E.] Wool" (Thompson 1997: 12). The condition of the enlisted soldiers' barracks and camps figures prominently in Army correspondence from the late nineteenth to early twentieth centuries. Temporary camps and barracks buildings were continuously constructed and reconstructed to accommodate the regiments stationed at the post. During the Spanish-American War of 1898, the Presidio hosted 11 to 41 officers and 231 to 872 enlisted men of the 4th Cavalry (Thompson 1997: 255). The first volunteer troops arrived at the Presidio in June 1898. A larger number of volunteer troops, nearly all infantry, also set up camp to the south of the Presidio at Camp Merritt, which was described as "unhealthy, ill-drained, and wind-swept" (Thompson 1997: 256). When the War Department ordered the formation of the 8th Army Corps for service in the Philippine Islands, 22,000 men occupied Camp Merritt at the Presidio (Thompson 1997: 276).

In 1890, permanent brick buildings had been constructed on Montgomery Street, also known as "infantry row" (Thompson 1997). The barracks were built to consolidate troops after many of the frontier posts were closed. They also provided a more healthful living arrangement than the camps that were scattered across the Presidio post. The barracks, built in the Colonial Revival style, were some of the first in the United States to be constructed out of brick. Each of the barracks buildings had a kitchen, mess hall, and common area on the first floor, with sleeping quarters on the third floor (Thompson 1997). War Department regulations required that all barracks occupied by their organization were properly ventilated, heated, lighted, kept clean, and in sanitary condition at all times (Harvard 1909: 40). Company commanders were to ensure that all beds and furniture were in good order, and that the same went for all public property in possession of enlisted men (Harvard 1909: 41). Each of the barracks could accommodate a company of 110 soldiers. It is not known which specific companies were housed in the Montgomery Street Barracks from 1890 until after World War II. At the end of the nineteenth century and beginning of the twentieth, the segregated, all-Black 9th Cavalry and 24th Infantry were garrisoned at the Presidio. The 9th Cavalry may have stayed in the Montgomery Street Barracks, or they may have occupied the older Civil War–era barracks on the post (Thompson 1997).

Under the aegis of the Presidio Trust, this project focuses on artifacts recovered from one of the Montgomery Street Barracks buildings, Presidio Building 104 (Figure 5.3), which currently serves as the Walt Disney Museum. In 2008, plant construction crews began rehabilitation work on Building 104. During the early phases of work, crews came across collections of historic-period materials in the eaves of the building. Presidio archaeologists subsequently retrieved nearly sixty boxes of objects from the building during rehabilitation phases. The majority of the objects in the Building 104 collection were retrieved from niches between the eaves, architectural features known as "soffit boxes." Scaffolding set up around the exterior of the building allowed archaeologists to access the eaves from the exterior of the third floor. Historically, soldiers on the third floor would have been able to reach the soffit boxes from the interior. In later periods, boards were nailed over the niches to close off the soffit boxes, thus securing their contents. In 2008, archaeologists mapped and removed the contents of each of the boxes. There is no indication from the field notes that archaeologists were able to discern distinct depositional episodes or temporal sequences in the boxes. After the object recovery phases of the

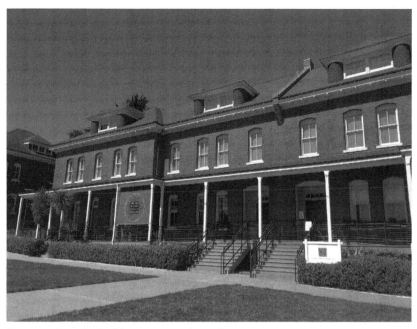

Figure 5.3. Presidio Building 104, now the Walt Disney Museum.

project, objects were sorted in the Presidio Archaeology Lab and housed for storage.

In 2018, in collaboration with the Presidio Trust and heritage staff, I developed a research project to study artifacts recovered from Building 104. My broader goals were to examine turn-of-the-century healthcare-related objects from the barracks in relation to their broader sociopolitical contexts. Progressive Era reforms of the early 1900s had a direct impact on the way in which military medicine was practiced and how soldiers viewed their bodies and health in relation to broader discourses concerning responsibility and national belonging. Studying the objects retrieved from Building 104 helps us to understand these dynamics.

Eighty percent of the paper items, including newspapers, blue books, coupons, business cards, and insurance paperwork, could be assigned to a particular year or decade, with dates clustering between the 1910s and 1920s. All the dateable objects in the collection were dated using trademark information, maker's marks, patent information, manufacturing method, or dates printed on the items. The earliest-dated object is a box of Colgate's Ribbon Dental Cream from 1896, while the latest-dated object is from

1945, a laundry receipt for a soldier of the 2nd Italian Quartermaster's Service Company. The most common artifact type (by weight and count) from the assemblage is paper, such as wrapping, newspaper, business cards, letters, and miscellaneous unprinted paper. Glass was the second most frequent artifact type (also by weight and count) and includes alcohol bottles, soda bottles, shoe polish, and hygiene and medicine bottles. Objects such as food and candy wrappers, rosaries, textbooks, personal letters, product information inserts, and business cards were also found. Military-related items include paper targets, military manuals, cartridges, uniforms and clothing items, and informational booklets. Healthcare and recreational drug-related items include alcohol and medicine bottles, tobacco products, toothpaste, dental floss, OTC medicine boxes, soap wrappers, and razor blades and packaging.

The Building 104 assemblage is significant for several reasons. It contains ephemeral objects not typically found in archaeological contexts; papers and textiles are remarkably common in the Building 104 assemblage. This provides researchers a unique opportunity to conduct archival research alongside more traditional archaeological kinds of investigations. Because of the individual nature of the finds, the collection provides a rare opportunity to explore the military experience. The assemblage includes items that suggest how individuals spent their free time, as indicated by pencil drawings, reminder notes, movie ticket stubs, business cards for local hotels and bars, and small collections of polished rocks and seashells, presumably from nearby beaches. It is clear from the context of the finds that some, if not many, of the items may have been intentionally curated or cached by enlisted soldiers. The soffit boxes were accessible from inside the third floor of the dormitories but would not have been visible during Sunday room inspections. While the soffit boxes may have served as a convenient disposal spot for chewing gum, paper wrappers, and food detritus, they also provided a safe space for storing personal or even contraband items.

Finally, research on the US military occupies an ambivalent space within the discipline of archaeology. North American archaeological investigations of military installations are overwhelmingly focused on impermanent conflict locations such as battlefields, genocide sites, or forts and encampments (Geier et al. 2014; Hanson 2019; Scott and McFeaters 2011; Starbuck 2011; Steele 2008). Unlike our Latin American and Spanish counterparts (Funari et al. 2009; González Ruibal 2020), North American archaeologists seem more reticent to seriously confront the long-term, quotidian, and often discomforting histories of US military contexts, including twentieth-century militarism, nationalism, technoscience, the complex intersections between military and civilian life, and the economic and psychosocial precarity of many contemporary military veterans. Histories of enlisted men tend to oversimplify their motivations and unique experiences by treating enlistment as an imperialist venture guided by a "desire to enforce Western policies" (Wilkie 2019: 129). Rather than assume the nationalist and imperialist motivations of enlisted men at the Presidio of San Francisco, I aimed to examine their quotidian experiences, a subject of study that remains lacking in historical archaeological scholarship. As such, I considered how consumer items became a means by which citizenship ideals were asserted and reconfigured in daily practice (Camp 2011).

Personal Hygiene-Related Objects

Several hygiene objects were recovered from Building 104. These include Palmolive soap wrappers, Pinaud Elixir Shampoo, Eau de Quinine Pinaud Hair Tonic, Colgate toothpaste, dental floss, Cutex Cuticle Oil, Gillette razors, and Chesebrough petroleum jelly.

Eau de Quinine hair products were introduced in the 1850s by Edouard Pinaud, a Paris-based perfumery (National Museum of American History, n.d.). Quinine was popularized as an antimalarial drug during the mid-nineteenth century and was often prescribed to domestic troops (Ockenhouse et al. 2005); it was also used "off-label" in hygiene products by the late 1890s. When heavily diluted in hair products, quinine was thought to mitigate hair loss (National Museum of American History, n.d.). Quinine was a key ingredient in hair care produced by Pinaud. Pinaud's shampoo and hair tonics were sold into the 1960s and were lauded as the official hair products of James Bond during the latter half of the twentieth century (Storey 2011).

The assemblage also includes seven boxes and product inserts for Colgate toothpaste (Figure 5.4). The company was founded in 1806 by William Colgate (Lippert 2013). It initially produced starch, candles, and soap, but after the company was transferred to Samuel Colgate, Colgate & Company developed an antiseptic dental powder in 1870 and began producing dental paste in 1896 (Colgate-Palmolive 2024). The Colgate packages at the Presidio date to the late 1890s, with the exception of one package that dates to 1927.

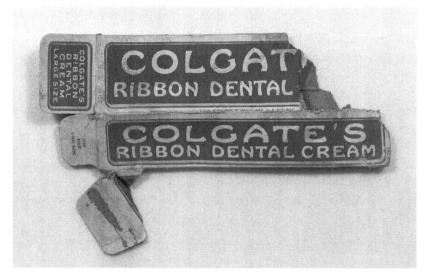

Figure 5.4. Colgate Ribbon Dental Cream box from Building 104.

Items for hand and nail care from Building 104 include Cutex Cuticle Oil and a pink bottle of Cutex Nail Color. Northam Warren Corporation created Cutex in 1916 (Forde 2002). During the 1920s and 1930s, cuticle care products and nail color predominately targeted middle-class women through advertising campaigns (Forde 2002).

Gillette razor blades and blade packages were also recovered from Building 104. The Gillette Company was founded in 1901 by King Camp Gillette (Oldstone-Moore 2015). By the late 1800s, men's facial hair trends were quickly changing; long beards were no longer fashionable and cleanly shaven cheeks and trimmed mustaches were in fashion (Oldstone-Moore 2015). While men could go to a barber once or twice a week, Gillette and his business partner, William Nickerson, developed a flat, double-edged razor blade that could be safely used at home (Oldstone-Moore 2015). Production of Gillette safety razors began in 1903 (Procter & Gamble 2023).

Finally, a small jar of Chesebrough petroleum jelly was recovered from Building 104. Two fragments of Vaseline wrappers were also found in the same context. The Chesebrough Manufacturing Company was founded in 1859 by Robert Chesebrough; an oil company, it also produced petroleum jelly, or Vaseline (Jayakumar and Micheletti 2017). Petroleum jelly was advertised as a cosmetic skin product, a skin moisturizer, and a healing ointment for cuts and burns (Jayakumar and Micheletti 2017).

Pharmaceuticals and Social Hygiene Items

Pharmaceuticals from Building 104 include Knoxit Injection, Larkspur Lotion, Sloan's Family Liniment, Ex-Lax, and Smith Brothers Cough Drops (Figure 5.5).

Knoxit Globules and Knoxit Injection creams were produced by Beggs Manufacturing Company in Chicago from the 1860s until the 1920s. Beggs sold remedies such as Beggs Hair Renewer, Beggs Royal Tooth Soap, Beggs Blood Purifier and Blood Maker, and Beggs Dandelion Bitters. From 1918–

Table 5.1. Artifacts from Building 104

Count	Object Description
Personal Hygiene Objects	
15	Soap wrapper (Colgate Palmolive-Peet, Palmolive, Ivory, LUX)
2	Palmolive-Peet Company, the Palmolive-Peet Company product insert
1	Pinaud Elixir Shampoo bottle
1	Eau de Quinine Pinaud Hair Tonic bottle
2	Pinaud's Shampoo product insert
3	Hygiene of the Scalp Compound Hair Tonic product label
6	Colgate's Ribbon Dental Cream box
1	Colgate's Dental Cream insert
10	Dental floss fragments (string)
3	Cutex Cuticle Oil package
6	Cutex Cuticle Cream product insert
1	Cutex Nail Polish bottle
5	Gillette razor blade packaging
14	Disposable alloy razor blade
4	Chesebrough MFG Company Vaseline box
2	Vaseline brand package
Pharmaceuticals and Social Hygiene Objects	
1	Knoxit Injection bottle
1	Venereal disease informational pamphlet (United Health Services)
1	Larkspur Lotion bottle
1	August 1928 package, calendar, advertisement for Sloan's Family Liniment
1	Nyal Cough Medicine bottle
1	Ex-Lax container
1	Smith's Cough Drops box
Recreational Drugs	
11	Flask (bottle)
59	Cigarette butt
20	Cigarette package (Chesterfield, Camel)

1919, federal authorities seized a number of nostrums that were said to treat venereal diseases, including Knoxit Injections (United States Food and Drug Administration 1920: 201). In 1919, chemical analyses of Knoxit by the Bureau of Chemistry showed that the solution contained zinc acetate, glycerine, and water, perfumed with oil of rose. The product was declared misbranded since it was falsely and fraudulently represented as a cure for gonorrhea. Because of the fraudulent claims made by the manufacturers, the District of California filed lawsuits and forfeitures in 1919, and the company was subject to legal judgments in 1920.

Larkspur Lotion was made by the Hance Brothers and White Company. The bottle's label claims that it is "effective in destroying head and crab lice: for external use only" (Figure 5.6). The active ingredients included alkaloids, acetone, acetic acid, and alcohol (10 percent). The bottle found at the Presidio likely dates to the early 1900s.

The bottle of Sloan's Family Liniment also dates to the early 1900s. Sloan's Family Liniment was produced by Dr. Earl S. Sloan after the Civil War. The label on the bottle states, "Externally: Recommended by us in the treatment of Muscular Congestion and Muscular Cramps due to exposure and fatigue, Sprains and Strains of Muscles and Tendons, Neuralgia from exposures and drafts, Bruises, Frostbites, Mosquito Bites. AN EXCELLENT COUNTER-IRRITANT."

Ex-Lax was invented by a Hungarian-born pharmacist, Max Kiss, in 1906. By 1926, Ex-Lax was the most popular OTC laxative in the United States. A chemical report from 1916 indicates that Ex-Lax contained water, phenolphthalein, ash, sucrose, starch, and chocolate.

Smith Brothers Cough Drops were branded in 1847 by James Smith, who owned a sweets shop in New York. In 1866, James's sons, William and Andrew, took over the company. The cough drops claimed to treat hoarseness, coughs, and sore throat. A chemical report from 1913 indicates that the cough drops contained sugar, charcoal, and sassafras flavoring.

Recreational Drugs

Recreational drug-related artifacts from Building 104 include cigarette butts, cigarette packaging and tobacco bags, and glass alcohol bottles and flasks.

The collection includes fifty-nine used (smoked) cigarette butts. The butts include both Chesterfield and Camel brand cigarettes, as well as unidentifiable, unmarked cigarettes. Cigarette packaging includes eighteen complete and fragmented packages for both Chesterfield and Camel ciga-

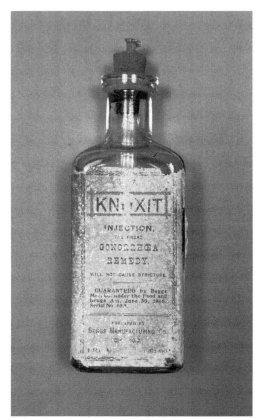

Figure 5.5. Knoxit Injection bottle from Building 104.

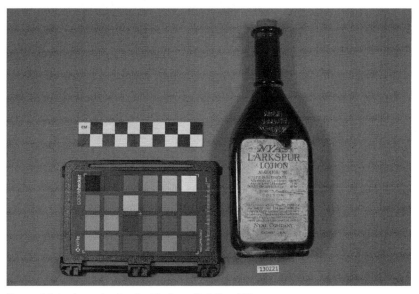

Figure 5.6. Larkspur Lotion bottle from Building 104.

rettes. The St. Louis, Missouri-based Drummond Tobacco Company introduced the Chesterfield brand cigarettes in 1873. The R.J. Reynolds Tobacco Company first produced Camel cigarettes in 1913. Reynolds revolutionized tobacco smoking with pre-rolled cigarettes. Camel cigarettes included a blend of several types of tobacco rolled in Turkish paper, an imitation of the Egyptian cigarettes that were fashionable during the early twentieth century.

Alcohol bottles from Building 104 include six glass flask-shape bottles and three square glass bottles. None of the bottles include paper labels or embossing. Based on maker's marks and/or manufacturing methods, the bottles date from the 1890s to 1929. Five of the flask-shape bottles have cork stoppers in the neck. One of the square bottles contains a gold-colored vitreous fluid.

Discussion

The material remains recovered from the Montgomery Street Barracks can provide insights into how health concerns and ideals concerning moral biocitizenship were entangled with daily life for soldiers at the Presidio. Individuals at the Presidio who confronted daily health challenges necessarily negotiated the Army's terms of health and biocitizenship (Epstein 2018: 23). By focusing on hygiene products, medicines, and recreational drugs from the barracks, we can examine how soldiers navigated issues of biocitizenship, bodily care, and medical authority in their everyday lives. Importantly, many of these individuals may have provided care for themselves in ways that diverged from the expectations of the US Army Medical Department, War Department, and commanding officers.

It is difficult to state with certainty what the discard behaviors at the Presidio barracks indicate—whether the eaves provided a convenient disposal location for everyday waste, or whether specific items were intentionally hidden in these spaces. One point in favor of the latter interpretation is that Sunday room inspections were mandatory and any prohibited item or object out of place was cause for reprimand, which usually meant suspension of Sunday leave from the post (Woodhull 1890: 40). In addition, some of the objects found at the Presidio represent items that the US Army explicitly banned for soldiers' use: liquor consumption, certain OTC medications, and even smoking tobacco in the barracks were forbidden. As such, this study intersects with other archaeological research that focuses on clandestine, hidden, or shadow economies (Casella 2000; Hartnett and Dawdy 2013, Yamin and Seifert 2023).

Perhaps most closely analogous to the Presidio study is Bryant and colleagues' (2020) examination of concealed objects from a mental health institution, the Royal Derwent Hospital in Tasmania. The Derwent Hospital project focuses on more than 1,000 pieces of ephemera cached below the veranda of a nineteenth- and twentieth-century asylum ward for middle-class women. Like the Presidio collection, the Derwent Hospital collection also includes items not typically found in archaeological excavations, such as clothing, documents, books, food packaging, letters, and other ephemera. Other items include carefully wrapped "bundles" embroidered with motifs (Bryant et al. 2020). While there are obvious historical and contextual differences between the Derwent Hospital and the Presidio barracks, the locations of the finds, the likelihood of caching behavior, and the types of materials recovered are similar. And as the authors of the Derwent Hospital study argue, the particular context of the items presents opportunities for researchers to study them taphonomically and archaeologically, but "also as a 'collection' curated by an actor within a unique set of circumstances" (Bryant et al. 2020: 169). The authors note, "What emerges is . . . an assemblage of small, ordinary things, often not valued archaeologically for their potential to throw light on either personal biographies or larger historical narratives, but which in this case constitute a vivid material 'underlife' that is seldom encountered" (Bryant et al. 2020: 169). The assemblage from Building 104 similarly represents a material "underlife" of soldiers posted at the Presidio during the Progressive Era. This provides invaluable information concerning how soldiers practiced self-care within the broader institutional guidelines and regulations of the US Army. While preventative care and curative strategies are often practiced in private settings, they reflect broader social and political circumstances (Ryzewski 2007).

Personal Hygiene and Care

All US Army personnel were expected to maintain strict standards of hygiene, including personal cleanliness and keeping their surroundings clean. During the late nineteenth and early twentieth century, the Army published medical manuals that detailed standards of hygiene, exercise, food, water, and general behavior. Medical Corps physicians wrote the medical manuals, which were primarily intended for medical officers and line and staff officers who were in command of troops. These educational manuals included chapters on infectious diseases, parasitic diseases, "diseases caused by immoral and intemperate habits," exercise, personal hygiene, and food and water (Harvard 1909; Woodhull 1890). One such manual, published in 1909, was recovered from Building 104: *Military Hygiene for the Military Services of the United States* by Valerie Harvard, MD (Harvard 1909). The manual offers detailed information concerning standards of hygiene that troops implemented and commanding officers enforced. Daily hygiene practices were to include bathing the body with soap, toothbrushing, face shaving, and keeping toe- and fingernails clean and short (Harvard 1909). If soldiers were infected with skin parasites, including lice, they were isolated by the attendant officer and subject to "vigorous treatment" (Harvard 1909: 120).

Soap advertising and use has long been used to communicate ideas about disease, dirt, and cleanliness; it also has a long relationship with the regulation of the human body in terms of purity and citizenship (Smith 2008). In particular, soap has an extensive and controversial relationship with the racialized subject. Implicated in commodity racism during the Victorian era, soap invoked the alterity of colonized and racialized bodies. Advertising and distributing personal hygiene products, such as soap, was a way to colonize "other" bodies and bring them into the fold of civilization (McClintock 2005, 2013). Marketing soap in the colonies and at home to immigrant, racialized, and otherwise "othered" human bodies shored up the notion that filthy and unhygienic others had to be spiritually, physically, and morally cleansed (Wagner 2015). As McClintock (2013) argues, soap acquired a role in the quest for moral and economic salvation. With the advancement of germ theories of disease and innovations in public health, preventing disease could be managed through measures such as maintaining personal hygiene. Personal hygiene products took on a symbolic quality that went beyond cleansing as a physical act: "soap moulded morality with its inalienable quality as a quotidian cleaning technology" (Ibrahim 2020: 2).

Bodily cleanliness, in the form of the clean-shaven and washed body, was a focal point for Army medical officers (Woodbury and Moss 1918; Harvard 1909; Woodhull 1890). Army hygiene regulations promoted control over the body to achieve a healthy corpus and a pure character. Uncleanliness was linked to moral degeneracy and laziness, and also unnecessarily put the physical safety of soldiers at risk (Harvard 1909). The Preventative Medicine Division of the US Army included a Sanitation branch, which focused on both sanitation and preventative medicine (Simmons 1943). This branch officially developed in 1939, although it drew upon earlier standards of hygiene and sanitation (Simmons 1943); it was "dedicated to the study, development, and promotion of measures that would provide a healthful environment for soldiers" (Simmons 1943: 934). Evidently, Army standards and social norms about hygiene impacted soldiers living at the Presidio. Artifacts recovered from the Presidio barracks such as soap packaging, razor blades, shaving cream, and nail care products demonstrate that soldiers pursued personal cleanliness and hygiene, using popular brands of hygiene items that were available from the post store or pharmacies in San Francisco.

Dental Care

During the early part of the twentieth century, dental care and hygiene were a low priority for most Americans. While toothbrushes are often found at mid- to late nineteenth-century Chinese American sites, most groups neglected dental care (Hyson 2003). Tooth decay and gum disease were considered normal parts of life (Picard 2009). Archaeological studies from sites dating to the nineteenth and early twentieth century demonstrate that dental caries, tooth loss, and gum infection were common across all economic classes and age groups (Picard 2009). Military examination records also suggest high rates of tooth decay and loss among recruits. Examination records from 1909 indicate a standard of health that included six serviceable double bicuspid or molar teeth with at least two sets of opposing teeth on one side of the mouth and no fewer than one set on the other (Harvard 1909: 84). One-third of all Army applicants in 1909 failed to meet this standard (Picard 2009).

Dental hygiene and screening programs targeted children, particularly the children of immigrants since children were thought to be more easily assimilated into American life. During the 1910s and 1920s, dentists often emphasized that maximizing one's health and physical attributes would turn patients into better Americans (Picard 2009). For example, one dentist noted that "a number of the applicants are the children of our foreign population, [*sic*] we are helping to make them better citizens, better men and women" (Picard 2009: 19). Soldiers were similarly framed in paternalistic terms, as wards of the state and in need of bodily improvement. Soldiers' diseased gums and offensive breath were objects of critique by medical officers (Harvard 1909: 764). The most commonly recommended method of dental care was preventative, to keep the teeth clean and mouth "fresh" (Harvard 1909: 248); toothpowder and toothbrushes should be used daily.

Although dental flossing was not prescribed by military officers, the presence of dental floss in the Presidio collection is significant since flossing historically has been one of the most overlooked forms of dental care by patients (Bass 1948). "In cases where soldiers suffered from tooth decay, the care of the dentist must be sought" (Harvard 1909: 248). The presence of Colgate's Ribbon Dental Cream (toothpaste), dental floss, and written appointment cards for the post dental office indicates that soldiers at the Presidio participated in acts of dental hygiene.

Pharmaceuticals

Prior to the Pure Food and Drug Act of 1906, medicine companies were not subject to restrictions regarding labeling or contents (Conrad and Leiter 2008; Donohue 2006). Medicine companies stressed the importance of autonomy and self-medication through marketing campaigns designed to instill mistrust in the professional medical community (Conrad and Leiter 2008). The burgeoning advertising and patent medicine industry of the late nineteenth and early twentieth centuries influenced patients to think of their bodies in biomedical terms, while also spurring the development of a medical marketplace and a diverse therapeutic landscape (Donohue 2006). Citizens of the early twentieth century were faced with a plethora of available medications and a sense that self-treatment could democratize medical practice and turn passive patients into proactive "patient consumers" (Donohue 2006; Greene and Herzberg 2010). Not until the 1950s did the FDA regulate the manner in which drugs could be developed, advertised, and sold to the public (Donohue 2006).

At military posts like the Presidio, soldiers could obtain prescription medications either directly from Army medical personnel or from the post dispensary with a prescription (Thompson 1997). At the Presidio, they would have had access to prescription medications from physicians at the Letterman Hospital. OTC drugs could be purchased from the post dispensary or from local pharmacies in the city of San Francisco. Post dispensaries were required to keep records of any medications that were sold and any prescriptions that contained derivatives of alcohol, opiates, or coca leaves (Woodbury and Moss 1918: 247). The Army Medical Office was wary of the dangers of drug abuse and drug habits among enlisted soldiers. It strongly discouraged, or in some cases banned, self-medication by enlisted personnel, and took particular interest in education programs that would prevent self-medication, noting that "lectures, discipline, and the exercise of vigilance to bring culprits to justice and punish victims" were the only way to prevent patients' overuse of patent and OTC drugs (Woodbury and Moss 1918: 247). In cases where medical treatment was needed, enlisted soldiers were to report to their commanding officers, or directly to the Army hospital for care and treatment (Woodbury and Moss 1918). Medical texts indicate that soldiers were often thought to have been "hoodwinked" into buying OTC and patent medicines either to treat medical afflictions or for the temporary relief that many drugs offered. "Although soldiers get their medical attention and prescriptions for free, nevertheless, the more ignorant are sometimes beguiled into buying patent medicines and finding many of them to give transient pleasure, they continue to buy and become medicine tipplers" (Woodbury and Moss 1918: 153).

None of the products from Building 104 were likely used as substitutes for alcohol or as sedatives or painkillers, since none of the products contain sufficient quantities of alcohol or opiates to work in these ways. Instead, many of the products index bodily self-care. Knoxit Injection was marketed specifically as a cure for gonorrhea and did not have multiple uses, unlike many other patent medicines that could be used to treat a range of unrelated afflictions. While treatments for venereal diseases were readily available at Army posts in the form of hospital treatments and K-packs provided by officers, being diagnosed with venereal disease precipitated strict punishments. Self-treatment for venereal disease was a way for soldiers to avoid reprimands. The bottle of Larkspur Lotion similarly represents soldiers' methods of caring for the self in private: Larkspur Lotion was advertised as an insecticide for body and pubic lice, specifically. While soldiers were required to seek professional care for skin disorders, including lice, this would have also been an embarrassing situation.

Other OTC medicines include cough drops, liniment, and Ex-Lax stool softeners. These medicines indicate that solders were keen to mitigate chronic conditions such as coughs or throat pain, muscle soreness, and digestive troubles. Intestinal health became a primary concern for physicians and patients at the turn of the twentieth century. Medical professionals claimed that intestinal fecal decay caused bodily illness and that impacted colons would poison the body (Komara 2023: 167). Physicians frequently promoted "quick fixes" such as laxatives and purgative foods, including cereals, to maintain a healthy and "toxin-free" corpus. They also promoted longer-term lifestyle changes, such as daily exercise and good nutrition, to maintain intestinal wellness (Komara 2023). Importantly, soldiers were recommended by the Army Medical Department to "not get into the habit of using laxatives to keep the bowels open. Their continued use is injurious"; instead, soldiers should engage in "proper physical exercise" and eat ripe fruits and vegetables and cooked foods (Woodbury and Moss 1918: 152). The Ex-Lax packages from the Presidio suggest that soldiers were aware of societal discourses regarding colon health and used popular intestinal purgatives. The large number of All-Bran and Kellogg's Corn Flakes boxes from Building 104 may also allude to soldiers' concerns with intestinal health.

Alcohol and Recreational Drugs

During the early twentieth century, the Army Medical Department confronted what it saw as the related issues of alcohol use, sex, and immoral character. Soldiers were to abstain from alcohol, since "alcohol muddles the mind" and, in worst-case scenarios, its consumption could lead "straight to the brothel" (Woodbury and Moss 1918: 150). But alcohol had not always been banned on military posts. After the War of 1812, the US Army allowed sutlers, or traders, to sell nonmilitary-issue supplies on Army posts (Thompson 1997: 140). Sutlers could sell alcoholic beverages, and at the Presidio, they were encouraged to sell to soldiers in order to discourage them from frequenting neighborhood bars (Thompson 1997). However, in 1881, President Hayes banned alcohol sales by these sutlers on military establishments. At the Presidio, Angelo Berretta served as the sutler until 1890, when the secretary of war purchased his store and turned it into the post canteen (Thompson 1997: 241).

The prohibition of alcohol on base resulted in what the Army Medical Department feared would be the "growth of dens of dissipation and disease just beyond the jurisdiction of the commanding officer" (Gillet 1995: 49). The Army developed the canteen system in 1881 in an effort to manage and oversee its soldiers' recreational activities and keep them from straying into local bars, saloons, and other untoward establishments. Canteens sold only light beer and wine; the War Department viewed canteens as safe and moral spaces where enlisted soldiers could drink light alcoholic beverages, participate in wholesome recreational activities, and attend chaperoned parties (Baker 2016). Since the US Army owned and operated the canteens, there was greater oversight over soldiers' alcohol purchases (Baker 2016). But by 1898, the Army had launched various campaigns that promoted total abstinence from alcohol; by 1903, the Army Medical Department prohibited alcohol use by enlisted soldiers altogether (Baker 2016; Wintermute 2010: 189). In addition to alcohol, other social drugs like tobacco were similarly discouraged by the Army Medical Office. Tobacco was seen as an unhealthy habit since it increased "the work of the heart and . . . also takes away the sense of hunger or appetite" (Wintermute 2010: 151). The presence of flasks and tobacco products in the barracks indicates that soldiers defied Army expectations concerning reduced drinking or even complete abstinence from alcohol and tobacco.

Other forms of material culture indicate that soldiers commonly engaged in social activities outside the boundaries of the post. The receipts, coupons, and business cards from local San Francisco bars, hotels, and saloons found at the Presidio suggest that soldiers took part in drinking, dancing, and other social activities while off post. Using social drugs such as alcohol and tobacco while in the barracks or social settings may have been a form of self-medication for soldiers. Drinking alcohol could mitigate the stress of soldiering, act as an ameliorant for trauma, and provide a social activity that encouraged camaraderie among troops (Coffman 2009). Similarly, tobacco could temporarily reduce stress and enliven social relationships between users; it was even thought of as a powerful curative for lung disease by some medical professionals during the nineteenth and early twentieth centuries (Kell 1965). Thus, both alcohol and tobacco may have fulfilled myriad social and medical roles for soldiers at the Presidio, to include abating physical and psychological pain, diminishing boredom, and creating social bonds between soldiers.

Conclusion

Goods utilized in private, such as pharmaceuticals and hygiene products, are emblematic of the materialization of private and public identities. Both hygiene products and OTC drugs are essential to personal enhancement and "fashioning of the self" (Smith 2007): certain items like laxatives, intimate ointments, antifungals, and insecticide ointments are relegated to the private realm, and yet profoundly shape one's identity. By manipulating their bodies through the use of pharmaceuticals, hygiene products, and social drugs, soldiers located themselves within a sphere of moral biocitizenship and as people who took "personal responsibility for the care of oneself" (Halse 2012). By managing their bodies to meet the health and hygiene standards set by the US Army Medical Department and War Department, soldiers were able to associate themselves as members of a broader sociopolitical structure with access to certain rights. Attending to hygiene and medical care presupposed proper care of the self, which was essential for maintaining one's status as a member of the Army. It may also be the case that soldiers extended this space of moral biocitizenry to national belonging more generally. "Enlisted soldier" was the lowest rank in the US military, but enlistment also came with certain civic and political rights, which were especially appealing for immigrant communities. For immigrants, enlistment was not motivated necessarily by an overwhelming sense of nationalism but was rather grounded in a desire to secure these rights (Dragomir 2023). By participating in a medical field of practice with other soldiers, enlisted men at the Presidio referenced broader conditions of Army citizenship and US citizenship.

As a total institution, the US Army was designed to reshape the corporeal self, appearance, mentality, and sociality of soldiers (Coffman 2009). Admittance meant surrendering certain ways of understanding oneself, but it came with new privileges and responsibilities as well. Institutions, including military institutions, were also places that harbored an "underlife" of possibilities where individuals could negotiate and resist reconstructions of the self (Bryant et al. 2020: 169). Presidio soldiers' artifact stashing was a way of reconfiguring their private identities, along with resisting the Army institution that prioritized collective ownership (Casella 2007). The act of using, discarding, and caching objects associated with self-care helped to reconfigure one's self-identity at the Presidio barracks as both civilian and soldier. Self-care often maps onto or operates through "technologies of normalization" (Yates-Doerr 2012: 137), but definitions of self-care as biopower are insufficient for interpreting the intersubjectivity of care. There are multiple dimensions of self-care, including habit, histories of experience, bodily knowledge, communality, and differential material access. Soldiers' former experiences undoubtably shaped their affective engagement with certain self-care routines, while their former knowledge influenced the kinds of products that they chose to use.

Healthcare, hygiene, and social drug products recovered from the enlisted soldiers' quarters demonstrate how soldiers negotiated multiple, and often competing, logics of care (Mol 2008). While alcohol consumption and self-medication at the Presidio barracks may be viewed through the lens of noncompliance, or even deviance, decisions about how and when to medicate the self are grounded in one's perceptions of risk, the body, and self-fashioning. Individuals may resist viewing themselves specifically as *patients* with a medical condition and thus avoid medicating altogether (Smith 2007). In other instances, noncompliance references past experiences, medical knowledge, and intimate knowledge of the self. Alcohol consumption, the use of OTC medications, and self-treatment for venereal diseases were not simply ways of defying military regulations altogether. They were rather methods of performing moral biocitizenship and active membership in the Army in ways that made sense to *soldiers themselves* and also signposted military belonging, responsibility, and knowledge and care of the self.

As social scientists have noted, biopower is not merely control over life or a body, or a tool in the making of state power (Epstein 2018). While the Army Medical Department and War Department set the parameters of health governance, soldiers articulated alternative visions of health responsibility that referenced hybrid forms of sexual and physical health. Instead of framing soldiers' actions as patient compliance or noncompliance (resistance) to Medical and War Department norms, I suggest that the hygiene and healthcare objects from the Presidio were embedded within *different logics of care* (Mol 2008) that represented myriad acts of everyday "tinkering" (Mol et al. 2010: 13) and healthcare "tactics" (de Certeau 2013) on the part of soldiers. Although soldiers may have changed the rules of the game, they worked toward an endpoint of well-being. As Mol (2008) notes, self-care is a psychosocial response to life and a way of managing one's body based on experience and knowledge. Everyday self-care incorporates biomedical knowledge (acquired through advertising, medical literatures, and contact with medical professionals) and lay knowledge rooted in experience, which draws from pain management, habits and routine, and knowing "what works" (Mol 2008). Instead of focusing on the choice-making abilities of individuals, Mol suggests that we focus on what patients do and work to disentangle the messy ways individuals participate in their own care (Mol 2008: 8). Focusing on self-care also necessitates that researchers attend to the power dynamics between caregivers, institutions, and patients. By paying attention to small acts of care (including hygiene), archaeologists are well positioned to examine individuals' "social underlives" and how these small acts articulate with broader social and political norms.

6

Conclusion

Guiding themes in this book include the professionalization of medicine, medicalization and medical consumerism, and the broader relationships between power, agency, and healthcare institutions. By investigating these themes and drawing on the unique position of historical archaeology to illuminate the material instantiations of healthcare and medicine, we are better positioned to understand the past as well as the present. In doing so, we gain a richer understanding of the American experience and how medicine and care is disproportionately meted to its citizens. The following sections will discuss future directions in the archaeology of medicine and healthcare. Broadening the definition of care is a productive avenue for understanding the differential distribution of care and for exploring the relationships that develop in the clinical encounter.

Power and Agency in American Medical Practice: Professional Medicine and Alternative Therapies

A key leitmotif in this book is the relation of medical knowledge and practice to structures of power and authority. Within archaeological and historical research, medical knowledge and its application are frequently interpreted as tools of state oversight and administration. Chapter 5 demonstrates how the US Army mobilized specific definitions of physical health and hygiene that shaped civilian and military conditions of citizenship. "Biocitizenship" is a useful guiding concept that shows how the US Army Health Department understood soldiers' bodily health and hygiene as essential to military belonging. Soldiers' health and hygiene practices at the Presidio of San Francisco accorded with the Army's terms of biocitizenship, but also referenced specific methods of attaining health that often deviated from US military regulations. What it meant to be a "good citizen" also structured institutional care, as demonstrated by the archaeological and historical examples of tuberculosis sanatoria.

While these examples are obviously extreme illustrations of the connections between state power and bodily health, other examples in this book illustrate the more mundane, everyday intersections between macro-scale forms of power and healthcare. It is equally important for researchers to attend to the microscale; power, after all, is not all-encompassing but relational, and works through changing conditions of subjectivity and agency. Historical and archaeological examples in previous chapters show how patients' growing distrust of professional medicine and government oversight, in addition to emerging new medical marketplaces, shaped evolving consumer trends during the nineteenth century (Young 2015). The wide availability of proprietary drugs created a robust medical marketplace during this period that enabled patients to assuage their fears concerning institutional health oversight (Segal 2020). Finally, alternative systems of healthcare persisted despite efforts by both the professional medical community and the federal government to eradicate "quack" medicine. Archaeological research highlights the inequities of the professional field of medicine while also showcasing how communities developed and implemented alternative healthcare practices.

The historical archaeological studies summarized in this book provide important information regarding past medical technologies. This includes archaeological research concerning the expansion of scientific medicine via the development of new medical tools (Veit 1996) and medical educational programs in human anatomy and internal medicine (Halperin 2007; Hodge et al. 2017; Nystrom 2014, 2017). Archaeological studies highlight key historical moments in the professionalization of the medical field, including etiologies of disease, diagnosis, medical training and licensing, and treatment. Historical case studies show how university-educated physicians, the development of medical institutions like the AMA, state and federal reforms, and healthcare regulations have shaped the professionalization of American medicine since the late 1700s. Archaeological research has foregrounded the significance of the professional medical community's search for new medical technologies and diagnostics. For example, archaeological excavations at the former residences of physicians in New Brunswick, New Jersey, recovered medical apparatuses and implements used in surgery, including gynecological tools, hypodermic syringes, and general practice tools (Veit 1996). New medical technologies used in community practice contributed to medical science and hastened new developments in surgery and the broader medical field.

In addition to advancements in medical tools and technologies, anatomical dissection had a profound impact on medical knowledge and the professionalization and authority of the medical field. Although human dissection had been intermittently practiced in European and Euro-American contexts for centuries (Brenna 2021), dissection and anatomization did not become an accepted practice within the American medical community until the 1860s, when individual states passed laws regulating dissection as a branch of medical science (Richardson 2001). It is equally important to note that medical research has used racialized, classed, and gendered bodies in unethical and often traumatizing ways. The historical legacies of unethical treatment of marginalized people hasten negative health outcomes among these same groups and precipitate patient mistrust of clinical medicine today (Cooper Owens 2017; Savitt 1982; Washington 2006). Archaeological research on dissection and anatomization foregrounds the importance of studying the unethical foundations of medical practice and knowledge, the legacies of racist medicine in contemporary clinical practice, and the ethical requirements that guide the contemporary study of marginalized groups (Zuckerman, Kamnikar, and Mathena 2014).

As many of the case studies in this book demonstrate, medicine and healthcare cannot be divorced from their broader social and political milieus. Both scientific and nonscientific medical systems encompass cultural worldviews and ideologies, unique ontologies, and aspects of secular and religious thought. For example, Linn's (2008, 2010) research shows how Irish immigrants adapted key aspects of their medico-ritual practices in North American urban contexts. Linn's close reading of historical and archaeological contexts demonstrates how seemingly straightforward forms of material culture like soda water bottles took on new religious and medical significance for Irish American diaspora communities. The transnational character of health objects is also documented in African diaspora contexts, where patients and caregivers used market commodities in ways that imitated culturally familiar healthcare products. These examples indicate how healthcare often exceeds the strict limits of biomedical knowledge and scientific definitions of health. For many cultures, including Indigenous and diasporic communities, holistic healthcare treated the entire physical, emotional, mental, and community body. As archaeological research shows, healing practices among African American and Afro-Caribbean communities targeted the individual body-self and the social body (Scheper-Hughes and Lock 1987), which references one's relationship to nature, society, and culture (Mrozowski et al. 2008; Reifschneider and

Bardolph 2020; Wilkie 2000). African diasporic communities often created healthcare practices that included associations with the environment, they established community networks of care, and they formed healthcare frameworks that extended beyond narrow definitions of physical fitness (Lee 2017; Reifschneider 2018).

In discussing the professionalization of the medical field, this book simultaneously attends to "alternative" forms of medicine and therapeutic practice that fell outside the purview of scientific medicine. Case studies in this book demonstrate how alternative medicines offered patients agency over their bodies and their care. During the nineteenth and early twentieth centuries, proprietary medicines in particular provided an important source of self-medication for individuals who were excluded from seeking professional care by dint of their economic status or their social identity (Bonasera and Raymer 2001; Rotman 2010; White 2021). They were also widely used by patients who distrusted the professional medical community or felt excluded from professional medicine (Cabak et al. 1995). Other forms of alternative medicine found at archaeological sites included herbalism, hydropathy, and other popular forms of homeopathic practice (Linn 2010; Mrozowski et al. 2008). Identifying "alternative" modes of healthcare and healing in the archaeological record has been an important first step for archaeological studies of medicine and healthcare. Earlier, foundational studies in what may be called "medical archaeology" were overwhelmingly descriptive: they focused on counts and types of medicine bottles at archaeological sites, or they were analytical studies describing the contents of bottles from sites (Jones 1981, 1983). Other research perpetuated presentist and Eurocentric understandings of medicine as discrete, drug-based forms of treatment (Shaw and Sykes 2018). These interpretations of medical practice in the past tend to be reductive and ignore the rich bodies of evidence that indicate "alternative" (in other words, nonscientific and non-biomedical) ways of achieving well-being.

Recently, historical archaeologists have pushed for new interpretive approaches to healthcare and medicine by forging links between the medical humanities and clinical sciences. One of the effects of this change has been archaeologists' recognition of multiple ways of healing in the past and the acknowledgment that health-seeking behaviors are often entwined with culturally grounded attitudes toward food, the environment, the normative body, and what exactly constitutes well-being (Miller and Sykes 2016; Mrozowski et al. 2008; Reifschneider and Bardolph 2020; Shaw and Sykes 2018; Wilkie 1997, 2003). The epistemological divides between seemingly "different brands" of medicine might be productively questioned through the lens of disability theorizing within the discipline of archaeology. Recent work in archaeology focuses on the myriad ways in which ability is normalized through medical discourses, advertising, consumerism, affective responses, and personal experience (Camp et al. 2023). For example, ideologies of ability can be interpreted from the presence of certain patent medicine bottles that promised consumers a better quality of life, free from pain and disease. The ideology of ability (physical aptitudes, reproductive health, etc.) and the fear of disability (tiredness, aging, infirmity, etc.) shaped individual medical decisions that aimed to meet normative aspirations of health (Wilkie 2023). Even seemingly nonmedical technologies, such as window glass in tuberculosis sanatoria, were active agents in promoting normative understandings of health and well-being—in this case, an aspiration toward the absence of tuberculosis infection (Scott 2023). Institutions, including public health organizations and workplace programs, promoted specific health regimens that were grounded in specific ideologies of ability. Within formal institutions, "disability is foisted onto particular bodies, is understood as standing in opposition to ableism" (Wilkie 2023: 254), while influencing the kinds of medical interventions that are required. If material medical practices result from differing ideologies regarding ability/disability, then historical archaeologies are well positioned to address how different expectations and embodied experiences shape medical decision-making by institutions, agencies, and individuals. Furthermore, using "well-being" as an interpretive lens avoids some of the problematic binaries between abled/disabled (Surface-Evans 2023) and between biomedicine/folk/alternative medicine. Focusing on well-being allows archaeologists to see disabled bodies as happy and enjoying a sense of well-being, as well as broadening the interpretive scope of the archaeological record (Mrozowski et al. 2008; Surface-Evans 2023; Wilkie 2023).

Despite these important inroads, "finding" evidence of healthcare in the past can be fraught with methodological and interpretive challenges (Shaw and Sykes 2018). Exploring healthcare in the past offers archaeologists exciting opportunities to study diverse methods of treatments that deviate from our preconceived ideas about what care should look like archaeologically. Medical archaeology also encourages generative moments of self-reflection. It urges researchers to do holistic work, to use multiple bodies of evidence, to recognize our own biases concerning what medicine *should* look like archaeologically in order to explore diverse well-being practices in the past. For example, my own archaeological research at a Caribbean plantation hospital, a nineteenth-century Danish colonial period site in St. Croix, did not reveal the kinds of medical tools and techniques that dominated early scientific medicine (Reifschneider 2018). But this does not indicate an absence of healthcare at the hospital: instead, enslaved nurses and patients used local plant and animal resources to heal the "whole body" through ameliorative forms of care (Reifschneider and Bardolph 2020). Surface-Evans's (2023) work at McGulpin Point similarly encourages archaeologists to expand definitions of health and well-being, as well as what "counts" as care-related artifacts. Diverse objects including medicine bottles, smoking paraphernalia, hunting equipment, toys, and tea sets would have been used to support family well-being and happiness (Surface-Evans 2023). Noting the prevalence and importance of nontraditional forms of care and other objects that contribute to well-being encourages archaeologists to question narrow interpretive frameworks. Instead, they can recognize both alternative modes of healthcare and that the pursuit of well-being is culturally constructed and contextual, often permeating multiple facets of everyday life.

Future Directions: Toward an Integrated Medical Archaeology of the Past and Present

The historical and archaeological discussions in this book touch upon key developments in medical science and practice and demonstrate how historical archaeologists have contributed to our understanding of these decisive moments in American medicine. This archaeological research is important since many of these studies provide diachronic approaches to studying medical history while also focusing on the material and practice-based instantiations of healthcare. This body of work is also significant for shedding light on the contemporary American healthcare landscape. The inequities of the current American healthcare system are an outgrowth of the professionalization of the field of medicine, a widespread ethos of individualism, and marginalizing medical policies and practices that excluded certain communities from advantageous participation in the professional healthcare system (Baker et al. 2008; Matthew 2018; Singh et al. 2017). In addition, a long-standing legacy of medical experimentation on marginalized people in the name of medical science has led to a culture of distrust among racialized and otherwise marginalized communities (Cooper Owens 2017; Savitt 1982; Washington 2006).

Relatedly, many communities today use experimental, homeopathic, integrative, and other alternative forms of medicine. The widespread use of these alternatives helps to corroborate their presence and their importance in historical contexts. The identification of alternative medicine in historical and archaeological contexts, including herbalism and homeopathy, has been hampered by "post-Enlightenment preconceptions about what medicine actually *is*" (Shaw and Sykes 2018, emphasis added). This is problematic since it renders traditional and alternative medicines in the past invisible archaeologically and serves to further delegitimize the importance of alternative medicine for contemporary practitioners. The goals of this conclusion section are not to argue for the validity or effectiveness of complementary and alternative medicines per se, but to show how contemporary health research on alternative healing and archaeological research on alternative medicine may be mutually informative. Research questions that span temporal periods and disciplines include *why* and *how* patients choose alternative medicine, and how neoliberal forms of governance and the logics of individualism underpin alternative forms of self-care *and* scientific mainstream medicine in similar ways.

The delegitimization of traditional and alternative medicine has a long history. Beginning in the fifteenth century, European administrators claimed that the traditional medicine practiced by Indigenous people was ineffective, "primitive," and/or dangerous. Delegitimizing the effectiveness and validity of traditional medicine in colonized territories was a crucial tool of European "civilizing" projects (Arnold 1993). European civilizing projects sought to colonize the minds and bodies of subjugated people through religious conversion programs, labor regimes, and alternate kinship structures, which directly impacted colonized peoples' medicinal practices (Anderson 1996, 2006; Arnold 1993). Anthropologists and sociologists have argued that similar language is used today by the professional medical community to describe patients' use of traditional medicine and alternative medicine as dangerous forms of pseudoscience (Eisenberg et al. 1998; Wootton 2005). Within European countries, Canada, and the United States, alternative medicine has become more accepted within mainstream medicine. There has been some acceptance of CAM in the US healthcare system as well, given that these care practices are sometimes covered by health benefit plans (McFarland et al. 2002). Ideological and practical reasons for this increased level of acceptance include structural factors like liability concerns, hospital protocols, and a general acceptance that they may offer psychosocial benefits to patients (Frenkel and Borkan 2003; Johnson et al. 2019; Sikand and Laken 1998).

Despite recent tolerance of alternative medicine and its integration into mainstream medicine, it is still often framed as resistance to and "opposite" scientific medicine; even the "alternative" in its name references its constitutive outside, in this case scientific biomedicine (Gale 2014). Since the late twentieth century, patients' use of alternative medicines has reflected broader sociopolitical shifts, including medical consumerism, feminism, and neoliberalism (Broom et al. 2014: 516). Sociologists and anthropologists have argued that the ascendency of neoliberal ideologies, which have permeated the professional medical field, has delegated responsibility for healthcare to the individual (Goldstein and Bowers 2015). Examples include prescription and OTC drug advertising, as well as public health promotions and biomedical campaigns that demand patients self-manage chronic conditions and infectious diseases (Lamb 2019; Sanabria 2015).

Within this political atmosphere, CAM use has been theorized as resistance to biomedical projects that place health responsibility with the individual patient. More recently, critical scholarship has questioned whether CAM and biomedical/scientific philosophies are truly divergent (Broom et al. 2014). These critiques ask how and to what extent alternative medicine similarly valorizes the individual subject and personal responsibility for health (Broom et al. 2014; McClean and Mitchell 2018). Alternative medicine ideologies often transfer health governance from the state to the self, such that CAM healthcare practices "may be contributing to the political shifts in governance and responsible citizenship that tend to fall under the rubric of 'neoliberalism'" (Broom et al. 2014: 516). In light of these critiques, both CAM and biomedicine reflect a similar predilection toward individual agency and autonomy in healthcare decision-making and healthcare practice. Ethnographic research by anthropologists and sociologists shows how CAM patients articulate aspirational health goals by relying on individual decision-making roles (Broom et al. 2014: 523). Furthermore, CAM use does not necessarily arise from limited access to biomedical healthcare. Because alternative practices seem to offer unlimited possibilities for healthcare opportunities, this seemingly allows users to take control over their health.

While the discussions in this section concerning alternative medicine use, neoliberal healthcare philosophies, and the destabilization of centralized forms of biomedicine have focused on the late twentieth century thus far, I end by arguing that archaeological research is well positioned to speak to these conversations. Future research can make significant and timely contributions on (a) histories of alternative medicine and philosophies of health governance, (b) the conceptual and practical boundaries between scientific and alternative medicine, and (c) the social, compassionate, and affective relationships that are enacted in medical encounters between healthcare providers and patients.

Regarding the first point, archaeology can destabilize scholars' claims that neoliberal philosophies of health governance have only recently influenced trends in scientific medicine and alternative medicine. Sociopolitical emphases on healthcare responsibility and individualism can be traced historically and archaeologically to at least the mid-nineteenth century. Healthcare responsibility discourses developed in tandem with political reforms that placed responsibility for health on the individual, alongside political discourses that blamed poor health on the "poor character" and habits of immigrant communities. Furthermore, a burgeoning and deregulated nineteenth-century pharmaceutical industry encouraged users to self-medicate to avoid the largely inaccessible professional medical field. Proprietary medicine production and use was technically deregulated until 1906; political discourses and marketing campaigns transformed ideas concerning patient choice and responsibility, which challenged the state's and medical community's responsibility for health.

Archaeological case studies focusing on proprietary medicine use have shown that these medicines gave patients control over their bodies and offered types of care not provided by the professional medical sector. Communities that were excluded from care, or that perceived themselves to be excluded from professional medicine, had a robust alternative medical market to aid them in achieving their health goals. In consideration of the preceding discussions, the question then becomes not *whether* alternative medicines offered patients agency and control over their bodies, but *how* and *to what effect* drug advertising, medicalization discourses, and patient-consumer decisions reflected a positive emphasis on individualism and choice. In light of this slightly different framing, archaeological research is well positioned to show how political discourses concerning self-governance warrant critical attention to tease out the relationships between patient choice, health responsibility, and health governance. This includes studying how alternative medicine values may have been entrenched in individualistic political philosophies. As such, archaeologists can enliven debates regarding the perceived differences between alternative medicine and scientific biomedicine, since both often encourage self-healing, self-responsibility, and self-care.

As many of the archaeological examples in this book show, culturally specific healing practices for Indigenous and African diasporic communities offered respite from political oversight (Cabak et al. 1995; Mrozowski et al. 2008; Reifschneider and Bardolph 2020). In this sense, culturally specific healing, religious/ritual care, and community-oriented healthcare may be considered emancipatory projects. But archaeologists must be careful not to overstate the extent to which people in the past had control over their health and well-being. Emphasizing patient choice regarding self-care risks de-emphasizing the wider environmental and occupational influences that degraded individual health statuses. Finally, it is important to recognize that *all* medicine philosophies often espouse health ideals that perpetuate unattainable health goals (Broom et al. 2014: 525). Contemporary critics have likened this relationship between healthcare aspirations and unattainability to Berlant's (2011) concept of cruel optimism. Cruel optimism refers to a relation to a thing that becomes sustaining, such that "a person or a world finds itself bound to a situation of profound threat that is, at the same time, profoundly confirming" (Berlant 2011: 2). Not all acts of self-medication may be interpreted as acts of empowerment, since self-care and self-medication may also entail an unending and unlikely search for better health "against the specter of its impossibility" (Berlant 2011).

Berlant's cruel optimism may be useful for considering how during the nineteenth and twentieth centuries, proprietary medicine companies intentionally overstated attainable health goals in their advertising campaigns, thus encouraging patients to constantly strive for good health by purchasing their products. Proprietary and patent medicines often claimed to treat a multitude of symptoms associated with industrial life and offered an alternative to treatments by physicians. Nineteenth-century patients could search through an unbounded field of therapeutic possibilities, especially since proprietary medicine companies recognized and perpetuated this unending search for good health (Young 2015). Future archaeological research may adopt a critical lens to examine how power and the sociopolitics of individual responsibility against the possibility of "good health" permeated fields of medical practice in the past. Given historical archaeologists' access to large and disparate bodies of evidence, as well as a unique ability to question the "modernness" of neoliberal forms of governance, future archaeological projects could ask: What kinds of common sociopolitical philosophies underwrite certain strains of medicine? How have the problematic logics of individualism perpetuated social inequalities in healthcare? How might both biomedicine and self-care articulate or reference certain forms of cruel optimism? How could historical archaeological research address these questions, and in doing so, foreground the importance of collective responsibility for healthcare? I believe that with its social justice bent, historical archaeology can provide examples of culturally sensitive models of collective care in the past that promote mutual responsibility and shared ownership of healthcare systems in the present.

In regard to the second point concerning the conceptual and practical boundaries between scientific and alternative medicine, archaeologists are also well situated to examine the complex intersections between different medical philosophies. Given historical archaeology's tendency toward scalar, bottom-up approaches (Gilchrist 2005), it is not surprising that archaeologists have approached alternative medical practices at the microscale. Archaeological research shows how patients selectively incorporated aspects of alternative therapies alongside professional medicine. Archaeological research on healthcare has focused on micro-level practices, in which patients and medical consumers may be described as "bricoleurs" who act within competing structures of health knowledge (Broom et al. 2014). The preponderance of alternative therapies in the United States can trace its roots to the purveyance of patent medicines, which the medical profession sought to curtail. Despite physicians' and the AMA's efforts to restrict nonorthodox medicine, patients and alternative healers continued to pursue herbalism, homeopathy, hydrotherapy, and other forms of alternative medicine.

Contemporary scholarship on CAM has interrogated the dichotomy between "orthodox" medicine (biomedicine) and CAM. This research often explores the "boundary work" that practitioners and patients undergo to maintain these distinctions (Brosnan et al. 2018). By studying everyday healthcare practices, research shows how human actors must continuously work to construct and maintain boundaries between different philosophical and practical divisions in medicine (Gale 2014). The practical and perceived boundaries between different categories or "orders" of healthcare practice have significant methodological and theoretical implications for historical archaeological research. In this dialogical, historical process, different biomedical and CAM modalities inevitably intersect and overlap. Historical research shows that despite the AMA's pejorative attitudes toward "quack" medicine, physicians frequently used herbal remedies and prescribed patent medicines because they were more effective or more appropriate. It is also unreasonable to expect that doctors always operated within the bounds of scientific reason and Western empiricism (Good 1993). Doctors' therapeutic choices are informed by personal experiences, the disease state of the patient, and the organizational structure in which they work (Good 1993). From a theoretical perspective, social science and clinical research often assumes the authority of scientific medicine, rather than demonstrating it. Scientific medicine is too easily reduced to a form of socially decontextualized practice without receiving the rigorous social and political analysis that "traditional" or alternative medicine receives (Vaughn 1991: 291). This a priori assumption perpetuates the idea that alternative medicine is a site of communal symbolism, while scientific medicine is a universal philosophy (Vaughn 1991).

Historical research on healthcare often complicates ontological boundaries between different veins of medical practice, as well as the socially and politically constituted nature of biomedicine. Future historical archaeological research can approach medical care as a dialogical process between conflicting but often intersecting healthcare philosophies, needs, and modes of expertise. Studying, for example, how physicians implemented medical training and knowledge in practice might require that archaeologists examine practices from the medical institutions or household settings in which they worked. Can we utilize the archaeological record to study the development of scientific medicine from a material culture perspective, and thus reach a more intimate understanding of diachronic changes in scientific medicine? Can we study spaces of clinical care, including spaces of medical training and practice, to explore the complex intersections between different medical systems?

Finally, historical archaeologists might critically examine the social relationships that are enacted in medical encounters between healthcare providers and patients. Can archaeologists, with the physical evidence we possess, study the entanglements and dependencies in medical encounters between provider and patient? Much of the historical research synthesized in this book focuses on patient self-care, or it considers the tools and techniques of early scientific medicine. Rarely have archaeologists interrogated the relationships between patients and providers, or the kinds of social and material worlds that are enacted in the medical encounter. Archaeologies of nonmedical institutions, such as asylums, almshouses, and reformatory institutions, may provide a helpful theoretical and methodological road map for studying the social and material interactions between provider and patient. How is medical care negotiated between provider and patient?

What kinds of larger power dynamics and institutional structures shape medical encounters? What are the affective relationships that arise in the medical encounter between caregiver and patient? Are historical archaeologists privy to these personal and often small-scale relationships?

These inquiries bring me to my final appeal for future archaeological investigations. As archaeologists and social scientists in related disciplines have argued, studying care practices is a way of making public what is usually delegated to the private sector. As Mol (2008) argues, disclosing the intimacies of care is a political act. If care practices "are not carefully attended to by research, they will be talked about in terms that are not appropriate to their specificities" (Mol 2008). Thus, researchers in all disciplines must be careful to consider the specificities of care and the work that both patients and caregivers do. Recent research in clinical medicine and the social sciences has argued that expanding the definition of *medicine* to *care* offers new interpretive challenges and opportunities. By focusing on care (instead of medicine), researchers are encouraged to think holistically about healthcare in the past; to move beyond research on specific tools and techniques of healthcare, such as surgery, hospital care, and medical interventions; and to consider all the components necessary for the maintenance of human well-being (Powell et al. 2017; Tilley and Schrenck 2017).

Importantly, care often involves compassion for impaired individuals who require assistance. Given the affective qualities of giving and receiving care, what if archaeologists look at medicine and healthcare through the lens of care, rather than biopower? What if bureaucratic institutions and administrative policies are not as totalizing as researchers have commonly assumed (Yates-Doerr 2012)? How might archaeologists investigate healthcare through multiple lenses that simultaneously recognize how care is inscribed by relations of power, but also note the "affections and moments of compassion" that are often enacted in intimate moments between patients and care providers (Mol 2008; Yates-Doerr 2012: 154)? While most of the archaeological examples and historical discussions in this book center around how political regimes of authority and precarity manifest in medical institutions and political regimes, archaeologists can also attend to the intersubjective spaces in which agency becomes distributed and shared (Hyde and Denyer Willis 2020). As medical anthropologists have been apt to point out in their own ethnographic work, care-in-action often entails practices and relationships that are incompletely described through analyses that foreground the importance of power (Yates-Doerr 2012).

While care is a recent concept in the discipline of archaeology, and it is widely debated whether emotion, affect, and care are amenable to archaeological investigation (Tarlow 2012), I nonetheless suggest that archaeologists have a social and political responsibility to search for those medical encounters that defy the regulatory poles of power and instead reference intimacy, empathy, and compassion (Yates-Doerr 2012: 139). I conclude this book by suggesting that archaeologists develop critical analyses of care that bypass the logics of power to enrich future studies of medical practice. Attending to the affective qualities of care, and its precariousness, encourages us to ask how caretaking illuminates the compromises and negotiations of those receiving and giving care.

REFERENCES

Abedi, Vida, Oluwaseyi Olulana, Venkatesh Avula, Durgesh Chaudhary, Ayesha Khan, Shima Shahjouei, Jiang Li, and Ramin Zand

2021   Racial, Economic, and Health Inequality and COVID-19 Infection in the United States. *Journal of Racial and Ethnic Health Disparities* 8(3): 732–742.

Abel, Emily K.

1997   Taking the Cure to the Poor: Patients' Responses to New York City's Tuberculosis Program, 1894 to 1918. *American Journal of Public Health* 87(11): 1808–1815.

2007   *Tuberculosis and the Politics of Exclusion: History of Public Health and Migration to Los Angeles.* Rutgers University Press, New Brunswick, New Jersey.

Adelson, Naomi

2000   *"Being Alive Well": Health and the Politics of Cree Well-Being.* University of Toronto Press, Toronto and Buffalo, New York.

Agarwal, Sabrina C.

2016   Bone Morphologies and Histories: Life Course Approaches in Bioarchaeology. *American Journal of Physical Anthropology* 159: 130–149.

Agarwal, Sabrina C., and Bonnie A. Glencross

2011   *Social Bioarchaeology.* Wiley, New York.

Ahmed, Syed M., Jeanne P. Lemkau, Nichol Nealeigh, and Barbara Mann

2001   Barriers to Healthcare Access in a Non-elderly Urban Poor American Population. *Health & Social Care in the Community* 9(6): 445–453.

Albanese, Catherine L.

1986   Physic and Metaphysic in Nineteenth-Century America: Medical Sectarians and Religious Healing. *Church History* 55(4): 489–502.

1993   *Nature Religion in America: From the Algonkian Indians to the New Age.* Chicago History of American Religion. University of Chicago Press, Chicago, Illinois.

Allen, Edward

1918   *Keeping Our Fighters Fit for War and After.* Century, New York.

Allen, Michelle Elizabeth

2008   *Cleansing the City: Sanitary Geographies in Victorian London.* Ohio University Press, Athens.

Amaya, Hector

2007   Dying American or the Violence of Citizenship: Latinos in Iraq. *Latino Studies* 5(1): 3–24.

American Social Hygiene Association

1918   *Keeping Fit to Fight*. War Department.

Anderson, Ann

2004   *Snake Oil, Hustlers and Hambones: The American Medicine Show*. McFarland, Jefferson, North Carolina.

Anderson, Gary M., Dennis Halcoussis, Linda Johnston, and Anton D. Lowenberg

2000   Regulatory Barriers to Entry in the Healthcare Industry: The Case of Alternative Medicine. *The Quarterly Review of Economics and Finance* 40(4): 485–502.

Anderson, Warwick

1996   Disease, Race, and Empire. *Bulletin of the History of Medicine* 70(1): 62–67.

2006   *Colonial Pathologies: American Tropical Medicine, Race, and Hygiene in the Philippines*. Duke University Press, Durham, North Carolina.

Antic, Tatjana, and Richard M. DeMay

2014   The Fascinating History of Urine Examination. *Journal of the American Society of Cytopathology* 3(2): 103–107.

Appel, Toby

2010   The Thomsonian Movement, the Regular Profession, and the State in Antebellum Connecticut: A Case Study of the Repeal of Early Medical Licensing Laws. *Journal of the History of Medicine and Allied Sciences* 65(2): 153–186.

Armelagos, George J., Peter J. Brown, and Bethany Turner

2005   Evolutionary, Historical and Political Economic Perspectives on Health and Disease. *Social Science & Medicine* 61(4): 755–765.

Arnold, David

1993   *Colonizing the Body: State Medicine and Epidemic Disease in Nineteenth-Century India*. University of California Press, Berkeley.

Ayo, Nike

2012   Understanding Health Promotion in a Neoliberal Climate and the Making of Health Conscious Citizens. *Critical Public Health* 22(1): 99–105.

Baker, Anni

2016   The Abolition of the U.S. Army Canteen, 1898–1914. *The Journal of Military History* 80: 697–724.

Baker, Robert B., Harriet A. Washington, Ololade Olakanmi, Todd L. Savitt, Elizabeth A. Jacobs, Eddie Hoover, and Matthew K. Wynia

2008   African American Physicians and Organized Medicine, 1846–1968: Origins of a Racial Divide. *JAMA* 300(3): 306–313.

Bambra, Clare, Ryan Riordan, John Ford, and Fiona Matthews

2020   The COVID-19 Pandemic and Health Inequalities. *Journal of Epidemiology and Community Health* 2020(74): 964–968.

Barnes, Jodi

2015   The Archeology of Health and Healing at Hollywood Plantation. *Drew County Historical Journal* 30: 18–27.

2021   Behind the Scenes of Hollywood: An Archaeology of Reproductive Oppression at the Intersections. *American Anthropologist* 123(1): 9–35.

2023 Tonics, Bitters, and Other Curatives: An Archaeology of Medicalization at Hollywood Plantation. *International Journal of Historical Archaeology* 27(1): 81–116.

Barnes, Patricia M., Eve Powell-Griner, Kim McFann, Richard L. Nahin

2004 Complementary and Alternative Medicine Use among Sdults: United States, 2002. *Seminars in Integrative Medicine* 2(2): 54–71.

Barr, Donald A.

2010 *Questioning the Premedical Paradigm: Enhancing Diversity in the Medical Profession a Century after the Flexner Report.* Johns Hopkins University Press, Baltimore, Maryland.

Barrett, Autumn R., and Michael L. Blakey

2011 Life Histories of Enslaved Africans in Colonial New York: A Bioarchaeological Study of the New York African Burial Ground. In *Social Bioarchaeology,* edited by Sabrina C. Agarwal and Bonnie A. Glencross, pp. 212–251. Wiley-Blackwell, Oxford.

Bashford, Alison

1998 *Purity and Pollution: Gender, Embodiment, and Victorian Medicine.* Macmillan, Basingstoke.

2002 At the Border: Contagion, Immigration, Nation. *Australian Historical Studies* 33(120): 344–358.

Bass, Charles

1948 The Optimum Characteristics of Dental Floss for Personal Oral Hygiene. *Dental Items of Interest:* 921–934.

Bates, Barbara

1992 *Bargaining for Life: A Social History of Tuberculosis, 1876–1938.* Studies in Health, Illness, and Caregiving in America. University of Pennsylvania Press, Philadelphia.

Bates, Donald G.

2000 Why Not Call Modern Medicine "Alternative"? *Perspectives in Biology and Medicine* 43(4): 502–518.

Baugher, Sherene

2009 Historical Overview of the Archaeology of Institutional Life. In *The Archaeology of Institutional Life,* edited by April M. Beisaw and James G. Gibb, pp. 5–13. University of Alabama Press, Tuscaloosa.

Beaudry, Mary C.

1993 Public Aesthetics Versus Personal Experience: Worker Health and Well-Being in 19th-Century Lowell, Massachusetts. *Historical Archaeology* 27(2): 90–105.

Beck, Andrew

2004 The Flexner Report and the Standardization of American Medical Education. *JAMA* 291(17): 2139–2140.

Beisaw, April M.

2016 Water for the City, Ruins for the Country: Archaeology of the New York City Watershed. *International Journal of Historical Archaeology* 20(3): 614–626.

Beisaw, April M., and James G. Gibb (editors)

2009   *The Archaeology of Institutional Life.* University of Alabama Press, Tuscaloosa.

Bendrey, Robin, and Debra Martin

2021   Zoonotic Diseases: New Directions in Human–Animal Pathology. *International Journal of Osteoarchaeology* (32): 548–552.

Berg, Manfred

2010   *Medicine and Modernity: Public Health and Medical Care in Nineteenth- and Twentieth-Century Germany.* Cambridge University Press, Cambridge.

Bergquist, Savannah, Thomas Otten, and Nick Sarich

2020   COVID-19 Pandemic in the United States. *Health Policy and Technology* 9(4): 623–638.

Berlant, Lauren

2011   *Cruel Optimism.* Duke University Press, Durham, North Carolina.

Berliner, Howard S.

1975   A Larger Perspective on the Flexner Report. *International Journal of Health Services* 5(4): 573–592.

Berman, Alex, and Michael A. Flannery

2001   *America's Botanico-Medical Movements: Vox Populi.* Pharmaceutical Products Press, New York.

Berridge, Virginia, Martin Gorsky, and Alex Mold

2011   *Public Health in History.* Understanding Public Health. McGraw-Hill/Open University Press, Maidenhead.

Betsinger, Tracy K., and Sharon N. DeWitte

2020   *The Bioarchaeology of Urbanization: The Biological, Demographic, and Social Consequences of Living in Cities.* Springer, New York.

Bevir, Mark

1999   Foucault, Power, and Institutions. *Political Studies* 47(2): 345–359.

Bishop, P. J.

1980   Evolution of the Stethoscope. *Journal of the Royal Society of Medicine* 73(6): 448–456.

Bivins, Roberta

2013   *Alternative Medicine?: A History.* Oxford University Press, Oxford.

Bivins, Roberta, Hilary Marland, and Nancy Tomes

2016   Histories of Medicine in the Household: Recovering Practice and "Reception." *Social History of Medicine* 29(4): 669–675.

Blakely, Robert L., and Judith M. Harrington (editors)

1997   *Bones in the Basement: Postmortem Racism in Nineteenth-Century Medical Training.* Smithsonian Institution Press, Washington, DC.

Blakey, Michael L.

2001   Bioarchaeology of the African Diaspora in the Americas: Its Origins and Scope. *Annual Review of Anthropology* 30(1): 387–422.

Blank, Robert H.

2012   Transformation of the US Healthcare System: Why Is Change So Difficult? *Current Sociology* 60(4): 415–426.

Blank, Robert H., Viola Desideria Burau, and Ellen Kuhlmann
2018   *Comparative Health Policy.* Bloomsbury, New York.
Blind, Eric Brandan, Barbara L. Voss, Sannie Kenton Osborn, and Leo R. Barker
2004   El Presidio de San Francisco: At the Edge of Empire. *Historical Archaeology* 38(3): 135–149.
Bonasera, Michael C., and Leslie Raymer
2001   Good for What Ails You: Medicinal Use at Five Points. *Historical Archaeology* 35(3): 49–66.
Bonderup, Gerda, Marie Nelson, Robert Jütte, and Motzi Eklöf
2001   Danish Society and Folk Healers. In *Historical Aspects of Unconventional Medicine,* edited by Marie Nelson, Robert Jütte, and Motzi Eklöf, pp. 76–77. Oxford University Press, Oxford.
Bos, Kirsten I., Kelly M. Harkins, Alexander Herbig, Mireia Coscolla, Nico Weber, Iñaki Comas, Stephen A. Forrest, et al.
2014   Pre-Columbian Mycobacterial Genomes Reveal Seals as a Source of New World Human Tuberculosis. *Nature* 514(7523): 494–497.
Bourdieu, Pierre
1977   *Outline of a Theory of Practice.* Cambridge University Press, Cambridge.
Bowleg, Lisa
2020   We're Not All in This Together: On COVID-19, Intersectionality, and Structural Inequality. *American Journal of Public Health* 110(7): 917–917.
Boyle, Eric W.
2013   *Quack Medicine: A History of Combating Health Fraud in Twentieth-Century America.* Healing Society: Disease, Medicine, and History. Praeger, Santa Barbara, California.
Bragdon, Kathleen J.
2017   Our Strange Garments: Cloth and Clothing among Native Elites in 17th Century New England. In *Foreign Objects: Rethinking Indigenous Consumption in American Archaeology,* edited by Craig Cipolla, pp. 110–126. University of Arizona Press, Tucson.
Brenna, Connor T. A.
2021   Post-Mortem Pedagogy: A Brief History of the Practice of Anatomical Dissection. *Rambam Maimonides Medical Journal* 12(1): e0008.
Brighton, Stephen
2005   An Historical Archaeology of the Irish Proletarian Diaspora: The Material Manifestations of Irish Identity in America, 1850–1910. PhD dissertation, Department of Anthropology, Boston University, Massachusetts.
Bristow, Nancy K.
1996   *Making Men Moral: Social Engineering during the Great War.* The American Social Experience Series 34. New York University Press, New York.
Broom, Alex, Carla Meurk, Jon Adams, and David Sibbritt
2014   My Health, My Responsibility? Complementary Medicine and Self (Health) Care. *Journal of Sociology* 50(4): 515–530.

Brosnan, Caragh, Pia Vuolanto, and Jenny-Ann Brodin Danell
2018   Introduction: Reconceptualising Complementary and Alternative Medicine as Knowledge Production and Social Transformation. In *Complementary and Alternative Medicine: Knowledge Production and Social Transformation,* edited by Caragh Brosnan, Pia Vuolanto, and Jenny-Ann Brodin Danell, pp. 1–29. Springer, Cham.

Brown, Kathleen M.
2009   *Foul Bodies: Cleanliness and the Making of the Modern Body.* Yale University Press, New Haven, Connecticut.

Brown, Philip
1911   The Opening of Arequipa Sanatorium. *San Francisco Chronicle,* 1911.
1914   Arequipa Sanatorium, A Sociological and Economic Experiment in the Care of Tuberculous Wage Earning Girls. *California State Journal of Medicine* 12(8): 327–329.
1919   The Subsequent History of Cases Discharged "Apparently Cured" from Arequipa Sanatorium for Wage Earning Women During Six Years. *American Review of Tuberculosis* 2(12): 764–771.

Brown, Tim, and Craig Duncan
2002   Placing Geographies of Public Health. *Area* 34(4): 361–369.

Bryant, Lauren, Heather Burke, Tracy Ireland, Lynley A. Wallis, and Chantal Wight
2020   Secret and Safe: The Underlife of Concealed Objects from the Royal Derwent Hospital, New Norfolk, Tasmania. *Journal of Social Archaeology* 20(2): 166–188.

Bryant, Vaughn M., and Richard G. Holloway
1983   The Role of Palynology in Archaeology. *Advances in Archaeological Method and Theory* (6): 191–224.

Buch, Elana D.
2014   Troubling Gifts of Care: Vulnerable Persons and Threatening Exchanges in Chicago's Home Care Industry. *Medical Anthropology Quarterly* 28(4): 599–615.
2015   Anthropology of Aging and Care. *Annual Review of Anthropology* 44(1): 277–293.

Bunton, Robin, and Alan Petersen (editors)
2002   *Foucault, Health and Medicine.* Routledge, New York.

Buzic, Ileana, and Valentina Giuffra
2020   The Paleopathological Evidence on the Origins of Human Tuberculosis: A Review. *Journal of Preventive Medicine and Hygiene* (61): E3–E8.

Buzon, Michele R., Phillip L. Walker, Francine Drayer Verhagen, and Susan L. Kerr
2005   Health and Disease in Nineteenth-Century San Francisco: Skeletal Evidence from a Forgotten Cemetery. *Historical Archaeology* 39(2): 1–15.

Bynum, Helen
2012   *Spitting Blood: The History of Tuberculosis.* Oxford University Press, Oxford.

Byrne, Katherine
2011   *Tuberculosis and the Victorian Literary Imagination.* Cambridge Studies in

Nineteenth-Century Literature and Culture 74. Cambridge University Press, Cambridge.

Cabak, Melanie A., Mark D. Groover, and Scott J. Wagers

1995 Health Care and the Wayman A.M.E. Church. *Historical Archaeology* 29(2): 55–76.

Cameron, Catherine M., Paul Kelton, and Alan C. Swedlund (editors)

2015 *Beyond Germs: Native Depopulation in North America.* Amerind Studies in Anthropology. University of Arizona Press, Tucson.

Camp, Stacey Lynn

2011 Consuming Citizenship? The Archaeology of Mexican Immigrant Ambivalence in Early Twentieth-Century Los Angeles. *International Journal of Historical Archaeology* 15(3): 305–328.

Camp, Stacey, Jodi Barnes, and Sarah Surface-Evans

2023 Special Issue: Health, Well-Being, and Ability in Archaeology. *International Journal of Historical Archaeology* 27(1): 1–266.

Camp Arequipa

2024 Camp Arequipa: Girl Scout Day Camp 2024. https://www.camparequipa.org/about/history.php.

Cantwell, Anne-Marie, and Diana diZerega Wall

2001 *Unearthing Gotham: The Archaeology of New York City.* Yale University Press, New Haven, Connecticut.

Capozzola, Christopher Joseph Nicodemus

2008 *Uncle Sam Wants You: World War I and the Making of the Modern American Citizen.* Oxford University Press, Oxford.

Carley, Caroline D.

1981 Historical and Archaeological Evidence of 19th Century Fever Epidemics and Medicine at Hudson's Bay Company's Fort Vancouver. *Historical Archaeology* 15(1): 19–35.

Casella, Eleanor Conlin

2000 "Doing Trade": A Sexual Economy of Nineteenth-Century Australian Female Convict Prisons. *World Archaeology* 32(2): 209–221.

2007 *The Archaeology of Institutional Confinement.* The American Experience in Archaeological Perspective. University Press of Florida, Gainesville.

Cayleff, Susan E.

1991 *Wash and Be Healed: The Water-Cure Movement and Women's Health.* Temple University Press, Philadelphia, Pennsylvania.

Chapman, Ellen, and Mark Kostro

2017 A Dissection at the Coffeehouse? The Performance of Anatomical Expertise in Colonial America. In *The Bioarchaeology of Dissection and Autopsy in the United States,* edited by Kenneth C. Nystrom, pp. 61–76. Springer, Cham.

Chatters, Linda M., Jeffrey S. Levin, and Christopher G. Ellison

1998 Public Health and Health Education in Faith Communities. *Health Education & Behavior* 25(6): 689–699.

Cipolla, Craig N. (editor)

2017   *Foreign Objects: Rethinking Indigenous Consumption in American Archaeology.* University of Arizona Press, Tucson.

Cirillo, Vincent J.

2004   *Bullets and Bacilli: The Spanish-American War and Military Medicine.* Rutgers University Press, New Brunswick, New Jersey.

Cisney, Vernon W., and Nicolae Morar (editors)

2016   *Biopower: Foucault and Beyond.* University of Chicago Press, Chicago, Illinois.

Coffman, Edward M.

2009   *Regulars: The American Army, 1898–1941.* Harvard University Press, Cambridge, Massachusetts.

Cohen, Ken

1998   Native American Medicine. *Alternative Therapies in Health and Medicine* 4(6): 45–57.

Colgate-Palmolive

2024   Our History. Colgate-Palmolive, https://www.colgatepalmolive.com/en-us/who-we-are/history, accessed February 6, 2024.

Condran, Gretchen A., and Eileen Crimmins-Gardner

1978   Public Health Measures and Mortality in U.S. Cities in the Late Nineteenth Century. *Human Ecology* 6(1): 27–54.

Condrau, Flurin (editor)

2010   *Tuberculosis Then and Now: Perspectives on the History of an Infectious Disease.* Associated Medical Services Studies in the History of Medicine, Health, and Society 35. McGill-Queen's University Press, Montreal.

Conrad, Peter

1992   Medicalization and Social Control. *Annual Review of Sociology* 18(1): 209–232.

Conrad, Peter, and Valerie Leiter

2008   From Lydia Pinkham to Queen Levitra: Direct-to-Consumer Advertising and Medicalisation. *Sociology of Health & Illness* 30(6): 825–838.

Cooke, Molly, David M. Irby, William Sullivan, and Kenneth M. Ludmerer

2006   American Medical Education 100 Years after the Flexner Report. Edited by Malcolm Cox and David M. Irby. *New England Journal of Medicine* 355(13): 1339–1344.

Cooper, Christine, Robert Fellner, Olivier Heubi, Frank Maixner, Albert Zink, and Sandra Lösch

2016   Tuberculosis in Early Medieval Switzerland—Osteological and Molecular Evidence. *Swiss Medical Weekly* 146 (0304): w14269.

Cooper Owens, Deirdre

2017   *Medical Bondage: Race, Gender, and the Origins of American Gynecology.* University of Georgia Press, Athens.

Cooter, Roger, and John V. Pickstone

2020   *Medicine in the Twentieth Century.* Routledge, New York.

Corbie-Smith, Giselle, Stephen B. Thomas, and Diane Marie M. St. George

2002   Distrust, Race, and Research. *Archives of Internal Medicine* 162(21): 2458.

Coveney, John

1998   The Government and Ethics of Health Promotion: The Importance of Michel Foucault. *Health Education Research* 13(3): 459–468.

Cowie, Sarah E.

2011   *The Plurality of Power.* Contributions to Global Historical Archaeology. Springer, New York.

Craddock, Susan

1995   Sewers and Scapegoats: Spatial Metaphors of Smallpox in Nineteenth Century San Francisco. *Social Science & Medicine* 41(7): 957–968.

1998   Tuberculosis, Tenements and the Epistemology of Neglect: San Francisco in the Nineteenth Century. *Ecumene* 5(1): 53–80.

1999   Embodying Place: Pathologizing Chinese and Chinatown in Nineteenth-Century San Francisco. *Antipode* 31(4): 351–371.

2000   *City of Plagues: Disease, Poverty, and Deviance in San Francisco.* University of Minnesota Press, Minneapolis.

2001   Engendered/Endangered: Women, Tuberculosis, and the Project of Citizenship. *Journal of Historical Geography* 27(3): 338–354.

Cramp, Arthur

1911   *Nostrums and Quackery and Pseudo-Medicine.* Vol. 1. Press of American Medical Association.

Creese, John L.

2017   Beyond Representation: Indigenous Economies of Affect in the Northeast Woodlands. In *Foreign Objects: Rethinking Indigenous Consumption in American Archaeology,* edited by Craig N. Cipolla, pp. 59–79. University of Arizona Press, Tucson.

Crossland, Zoë

2009   Of Clues and Signs: The Dead Body and Its Evidential Traces. *American Anthropologist* 111(1): 69–80.

Daniel, Thomas M., Joseph H. Bates, and Katharine A. Downes

2014   History of Tuberculosis. In *Tuberculosis,* edited by Barry R. Bloom, pp. 13–24. ASM Press, Washington, DC.

Day, Carolyn

2017   *Consumptive Chic: A History of Beauty, Fashion, and Disease.* Bloomsbury Academic, New York.

de Certeau, Michel

2013   *The Practice of Everyday Life.* University of California Press, Berkeley.

De Cunzo, Lu Ann

1995   Reform, Respite, Ritual: An Archaeology of Institutions; The Magdalen Society of Philadelphia, 1800–1850. *Historical Archaeology* 29(3): i–168.

2006   Exploring the Institution: Reform, Confinement, Social Change. In *Historical Archaeology,* edited by Martin Hall and Stephen Silliman, pp. 167–189. Blackwell Publishing, Malden, Massachusetts.

Deetz, James

2010   *In Small Things Forgotten: An Archaeology of Early American Life.* Anchor, New York.

de Klerk, Josien, and Eileen Moyer

2017   "A Body Like a Baby": Social Self-Care among Older People with Chronic HIV in Mombasa. *Medical Anthropology* 36(4): 305–318.

Delle, James A.

1998   *An Archaeology of Social Space: Analyzing Coffee Plantations in Jamaica's Blue Mountains.* Contributions to Global Historical Archaeology. Plenum Press, New York.

de Souza, Sheila M. F. Mendonça, Diana Maul de Carvalho, and Andrea Lessa

2003   Paleoepidemiology: Is There a Case to Answer? *Memórias do Instituto Oswaldo Cruz* 98(suppl. 1): 21–27.

Devine, Shauna

2014   *Learning from the Wounded: The Civil War and the Rise of American Medical Science.* University of North Carolina Press, Chapel Hill.

2016   "To Make Something Out of the Dying in This War": The Civil War and the Rise of American Medical Science. *The Journal of the Civil War Era* 6(2): 149–163.

DeWitte, Sharon N.

2016   Archaeological Evidence of Epidemics Can Inform Future Epidemics. *Annual Review of Anthropology* 45(1): 63–77.

Dickman, Samuel L., David U. Himmelstein, and Steffie Woolhandler

2017   Inequality and the Health-Care System in the USA. *The Lancet* 389(10077): 1431–1441.

Dincauze, Dena Ferran

2000   *Environmental Archaeology: Principles and Practice.* Cambridge University Press, Cambridge.

Donohue, Julie

2006   A History of Drug Advertising: The Evolving Roles of Consumers and Consumer Protection. *The Milbank Quarterly* 84(4): 659–699.

Donohue, Julie M., Marisa Cevasco, and Meredith B. Rosenthal

2007   A Decade of Direct-to-Consumer Advertising of Prescription Drugs. *New England Journal of Medicine* 357(7): 673–681.

Dormandy, Thomas

2000   *The White Death: A History of Tuberculosis.* New York University Press, New York.

Downey, Lynn

1994   "This Novel Employment of Untrained Hands": The Pottery of the Arequipa Sanatorium. *California History* 73(3): 202–215.

2019   *Arequipa Sanatorium: Life in California's Lung Resort for Women.* University of Oklahoma Press, Norman.

Downing, Sarah Jane

2012   *Beauty and Cosmetics, 1550–1950.* Bloomsbury Publishing, London.

Dragomir, Cristina-Ioana

2023   *Making the Immigrant Soldier: How Race, Ethnicity, Class, and Gender Intersect in the US Military.* University of Illinois Press, Urbana.

Duchêne, Sebastián, Simon Y. W. Ho, Ann G. Carmichael, Edward C. Holmes, and Hendrik Poinar

2020   The Recovery, Interpretation and Use of Ancient Pathogen Genomes. *Current Biology* 30(19): R1215–R1231.

Duffin, Jacalyn

2014   *To See with a Better Eye: A Life of R.T.H. Laennec.* Princeton University Press, Princeton, New Jersey.

Duffy, John

1993   *From Humors to Medical Science: A History of American Medicine.* 2nd ed. University of Illinois Press, Urbana.

Dunnavant, Justin

2017   Access Denied: African Americans and Access to End-of-Life Care in Nineteenth-Century Washington, DC. *Historical Archaeology* 51(1): 114–130.

Earnshaw, Valerie A., Lisa A. Eaton, Seth C. Kalichman, Natalie M. Brousseau, E. Carly Hill, and Annie B. Fox

2020   COVID-19 Conspiracy Beliefs, Health Behaviors, and Policy Support. *Translational Behavioral Medicine* 10(4): 850–856.

Eberl, Jakob-Moritz, Robert A. Huber, and Esther Greussing

2021   From Populism to the "Plandemic": Why Populists Believe in COVID-19 Conspiracies. *Journal of Elections, Public Opinion and Parties* 31(sup1): 272–284.

Eisenberg, David M., Roger B. Davis, Susan L. Ettner, Scott Appel, Sonja Wilkey, Maria Van Rompay, and Ronald C. Kessler

1998   Trends in Alternative Medicine Use in the United States, 1990–1997: Results of a Follow-up National Survey. *JAMA* 280(18): 1569.

Eisenberg, David M., Ronald C. Kessler, Cindy Foster, Frances E. Norlock, David R. Calkins, and Thomas L. Delbanco

1993   Unconventional Medicine in the United States—Prevalence, Costs, and Patterns of Use. *New England Journal of Medicine* 328(4): 246–252.

Epstein, Steven

2018   Governing Sexual Health: Bridging Biocitizenship and Sexual Citizenship. In *Biocitizenship: The Politics of Bodies, Governance, and Power,* edited by Kelly E. Happe, Jenell Johnson, and Marina Levina, pp. 21–50. New York University Press, New York.

Farmer, Paul

1996   Social Inequalities and Emerging Infectious Diseases. *Emerging Infectious Diseases* 2(4): 259–269.

2000   The Consumption of the Poor: Tuberculosis in the 21st Century. *Ethnography* 1(2): 183–216.

Fauci, Anthony S., H. Clifford Lane, and Robert R. Redfield

2020   Covid-19—Navigating the Uncharted. *New England Journal of Medicine* 382(13): 1268–1269.

Fillmore, Susan E.

1986   Samuel Thomson and His Effect on the American Health Care System. *Pharmacy in History* 28(4): 188–191.

Fisher, Charles L., Karl J. Reinhard, Matthew Kirk, and Justin DiVirgilio

2007   Privies and Parasites: The Archaeology of Health Conditions in Albany, New York. *Historical Archaeology* 41(4): 172–197.

Fitts, Robert

2001   The Rhetoric of Reform: The Five Points Missions and the Cult of Domesticity. *Historical Archaeology* 35(3): 115–132.

Flannery, Michael A.

2002   The Early Botanical Medical Movement as a Reflection of Life, Liberty, and Literacy in Jacksonian America. *Journal of the Medical Library Association* 90(4): 442–454.

Flexner, Abraham

1925   *Medical Education: A Comparative Study.* MacMillan, New York.

Ford, Nancy Gentile

2011   *Americans All! Foreign-Born Soldiers in World War I.* Texas A&M University Press, College Station.

Forde, Kate

2002   Celluloid Dreams: The Marketing of Cutex in America, 1916–1935. *Journal of Design History* 15(3): 175–189.

Foucault, Michel

1990   *The History of Sexuality: An Introduction.* Vintage Books, New York.

2010   *The Birth of Biopolitics: Lectures at the Collège de France, 1978–79.* 1st pbk. ed. [repr.]. Lectures at the Collège de France. Picador, New York.

Foucault, Michel, Paul Rabinow, and James D. Faubion

1997   *The Essential Works of Foucault, 1954–1984.* New Press, New York.

Fournié, Guillaume, Dirk U. Pfeiffer, and Robin Bendrey

2017   Early Animal Farming and Zoonotic Disease Dynamics: Modelling Brucellosis Transmission in Neolithic Goat Populations. *Royal Society Open Science* 4(2): 160943.

Franklin, Maria, and Samuel M. Wilson

2020   A Bioarchaeological Study of African American Health and Mortality in the Post-Emancipation U.S. South. *American Antiquity* 85(4): 652–675.

Frenkel, Moshe A., and Jeffrey M. Borkan

2003   An Approach for Integrating Complementary–Alternative Medicine into Primary Care. *Family Practice* 20(3): 324–332.

Funari, Pedro Paulo A., Andres Zarankin, and Melisa A. Salerno

2009   *Memories from Darkness: Archaeology of Repression and Resistance in Latin America.* Contributions to Global Historical Archaeology. Springer, New York.

Gabriel, Joseph M.

2014   *Medical Monopoly: Intellectual Property Rights and the Origins of the Modern Pharmaceutical Industry.* University of Chicago Press, Chicago, Illinois.

Gale, Nicola

2014   The Sociology of Traditional, Complementary and Alternative Medicine. *Sociology Compass* 8(6): 805–822.

Gamble, Lynn H., Cheryl Claassen, Jelmer W. Eerkens, Douglas J. Kennett, Patricia M. Lambert, Matthew J. Liebmann, Natasha Lyons, et al.

2021   Finding Archaeological Relevance during a Pandemic and What Comes After. *American Antiquity* 86(1): 2–22.

Gamble, Vanessa

1993   A Legacy of Distrust: African Americans and Medical Research. *American Journal of Preventive Medicine* 9(6): 35–38.

1997   Under the Shadow of Tuskegee: African Americans and Health Care. *American Journal of Public Health* 87(11): 1773–1778.

Geier, Clarence R., Douglas D. Scott, and Lawrence Edward Babits (editors)

2014   *From These Honored Dead: Historical Archaeology of the American Civil War.* University Press of Florida, Gainesville.

Gellad, Ziad F., and Kenneth W. Lyles

2007   Direct-to-Consumer Advertising of Pharmaceuticals. *The American Journal of Medicine* 120(6): 475–480.

Gibb, James G., and April M. Beisaw

2000   Learning Cast up from the Mire: Archaeological Investigations of Schoolhouses in the Northeastern United States. *Northeast Historical Archaeology* 29(1): 107–129.

Gilbert, Pamela K.

2004   *Mapping the Victorian Social Body.* State University of New York Press, Albany.

Gilchrist, Roberta

2005   Introduction: Scales and Voices in World Historical Archaeology. *World Archaeology* 37(3): 329–336.

Gillet, Mary

1995   *The Army Medical Department 1865–1917.* U.S. Army Center of Military History, Washington, DC.

Goldstein, Melissa M., and Daniel G. Bowers

2015   The Patient as Consumer: Empowerment or Commodification? Currents in Contemporary Bioethics. *Journal of Law, Medicine & Ethics* 43(1): 162–165.

González Ruibal, Alfredo

2020   *The Archaeology of the Spanish Civil War.* Routledge, New York.

Good, Byron

1993   *Medicine, Rationality and Experience: An Anthropological Perspective.* Cambridge University Press, Cambridge.

Graham, Elizabeth

1998   Mission Archaeology. *Annual Review of Anthropology* 27(1): 25–62.

Greene, Jeremy A., and David Herzberg

2010   Hidden in Plain Sight: Marketing Prescription Drugs to Consumers in the Twentieth Century. *American Journal of Public Health* 100(5): 793–803.

Greenhough, Beth

2014   Biopolitics and Biological Citizenship. In *The Wiley Blackwell Encyclopedia of Health, Illness, Behavior, and Society,* edited by William C. Cockerham, Robert Dingwall, and Stella Quah, pp. 145–148. Wiley-Blackwell, Chichester.

Guardino, Peter

2014   Gender, Soldiering, and Citizenship in the Mexican-American War of 1846–1848. *The American Historical Review* 119(1): 23–46.

Hall, M. and Silliman, Stephen W. (editors)

2009   *Historical Archaeology.* Blackwell Publishing, Malden.

Haller, John S.

1981   *American Medicine in Transition, 1840–1910.* University of Illinois Press, Urbana.

Halperin, Edward C.

2007   The Poor, the Black, and the Marginalized as the Source of Cadavers in United States Anatomical Education. *Clinical Anatomy* 20(5): 489–495.

Halse, Christine

2012   Bio-Citizenship: Virtue Discourses and the Birth of the Bio-Citizen. In *Biopolitics and the "Obesity Epidemic": Governing Bodies,* edited by Jan Wright, pp. 53–67. Routledge, New York.

Hanson, Todd A.

2019   *The Archaeology of the Cold War.* University Press of Florida, Gainesville.

Happe, Kelly E., Jenell M. Johnson, and Marina Levina (editors)

2018   *Biocitizenship: The Politics of Bodies, Governance, and Power.* New York University Press, New York.

Harley, Earl H.

2006   The Forgotten History of Defunct Black Medical Schools in the 19th and 20th Centuries and the Impact of the Flexner Report. *Journal of the National Medical Association* 98(9): 1425–1429.

Harley, Lilas, and Kathleen Barker Schwartz

2013   Philip King Brown and Arequipa Sanatorium: Early Occupational Therapy as Medical and Social Experiment. *The American Journal of Occupational Therapy* 67(2): 11–17.

Harrison, Faye V.

1994   Racial and Gender Inequalities in Health and Health Care. *Medical Anthropology Quarterly* 8(1): 90–95.

Harrison, Rodney

2002   Archaeology and the Colonial Encounter: Kimberley Spearpoints, Cultural Identity and Masculinity in the North of Australia. *Journal of Social Archaeology* 2(3): 352–377.

Harrod, Ryan P., and Debra L. Martin

2015   Bioarchaeological Case Studies of Slavery, Captivity, and Other Forms of Exploitation. In *The Archaeology of Slavery: A Comparative Approach to Captivity and Coercion,* edited by Lydia Wilson Marshall, pp. 41–63. Southern Illinois University Press, Carbondale.

Hartnett, Alexandra, and Shannon Lee Dawdy
2013   The Archaeology of Illegal and Illicit Economies. *Annual Review of Anthropology* 42(1): 37–51.

Harvard, Valerie
1909   *Manual of Military Hygiene for the Military Services of the United States.* W. Wood, Washington, DC.

Heath, Barbara J., Eleanor E. Breen, and Lori A. Lee (editors)
2017   *Material Worlds: Archaeology, Consumption, and the Road to Modernity.* Routledge/Taylor & Francis Group, New York.

Heffner, Sarah C.
2013   Exploring Healthcare Practices of the Lovelock Chinese: An Analysis and Interpretation of Medicinal Artifacts in the Lovelock Chinatown Collection. *Nevada Archaeologist* 26: 25–36.
2015   Exploring Health-Care Practices of Chinese Railroad Workers in North America. *Historical Archaeology* 49(1): 134–147.

Heller, R. F., T. D. Heller, and S. Pattison
2003   Putting the Public Back into Public Health. Part I. A Re-definition of Public Health. *Public Health* 117(1): 62–65.

Helman, Cecil G.
1978   Feed a Cold, Starve a Fever—Folk Models of Infection in an English Suburban Community, and Their Relation to Medical Treatment. *Culture, Medicine and Psychiatry* 2(2): 107–137.

Highet, Megan J.
2005   Body Snatching & Grave Robbing: Bodies for Science. *History and Anthropology* 16(4): 415–440.

Hodge, Christina J.
2013   Non-bodies of Knowledge: Anatomized Remains from the Holden Chapel Collection, Harvard University. *Journal of Social Archaeology* 13(1): 122–149.

Hodge, Christina J., Jane Lyden Rousseau, and Michèle E. Morgan
2017   Teachings of the Dead: The Archaeology of Anatomized Remains from Holden Chapel, Harvard University. In *The Bioarchaeology of Dissection and Autopsy in the United States,* edited by Kenneth C. Nystrom, pp. 115–142. Bioarchaeology and Social Theory. Springer, Cham.

Horton, Sarah, and Judith C. Barker
2009   "Stains" on Their Self-Discipline: Public Health, Hygiene, and the Disciplining of Undocumented Immigrant Parents in the Nation's Internal Borderlands. *American Ethnologist* 36(4): 784–798.

Hosek, Lauren, Alanna L. Warner-Smith, and Cristina C. Watson
2020   The Body Politic and the Citizen's Mouth: Oral Health and Dental Care in Nineteenth-Century Manhattan. *Historical Archaeology* 54(1): 138–159.

Howell, Joel D

2016   Early Clinical Use of the X-ray. *Transactions of the American Clinical and Climatological Association* 127: 341–349.

Howson, Jean E.

1993   The Archaeology of 19th-Century Health and Hygiene at the Sullivan Street Site, New York City. *Northeast Historical Archaeology* 22(1): 137–160.

Hoy, Suellen

1997   *Chasing Dirt: The American Pursuit of Cleanliness.* Oxford University Press, Oxford.

Hufthammer, Anne Karin, and Lars Walløe

2013   Rats Cannot Have Been Intermediate Hosts for *Yersinia pestis* During Medieval Plague Epidemics in Northern Europe. *Journal of Archaeological Science* 40(4): 1752–1759.

Hutchinson, Dale L.

2016   *Disease and Discrimination: Poverty and Pestilence in Colonial Atlantic America.* University Press of Florida, Gainesville.

2022   *American Health and Wellness in Archaeology and History.* University Press of Florida, Gainesville.

Hyde, Sandra Teresa, and Laurie Denyer Willis

2020   Balancing the Quotidian: Precarity, Care and Pace in Anthropology's Storytelling. *Medical Anthropology* 39(4): 297–304.

Hyson, John M.

2003   History of the Toothbrush. *Journal of the History of Dentistry* 51(2): 73–80.

Ibrahim, Yasmin

2020   Between Soap and Science: The Pandemic, Experts and Expendable Lives. *Social Sciences & Humanities Open* 2(1): 100080.

Institute of Medicine (US) Committee for the Study of the Future of Public Health

1988   *The Future of Public Health.* Vol. 88. National Academies Press, Washington, DC.

Institute of Medicine (US) Committee on Understanding and Eliminating Racial and Ethnic Disparities in Health Care

2002   *Unequal Treatment: Confronting Racial and Ethnic Disparities in Health Care.* National Academies Press, Washington, DC.

Jayakumar, Kishore L., and Robert G. Micheletti

2017   Robert Chesebrough and the Dermatologic Wonder of Petroleum Jelly. *JAMA Dermatology* 153(11): 1157.

Jenkins, Tracy H.

2020   An Intersectional Archaeology of Women's Reproductive Rights in Early Twentieth-Century Easton, Maryland. *Historical Archaeology* 54(3): 581–604.

Jensen, Niklas Thode

2012   *For the Health of the Enslaved: Slaves, Medicine and Power in the Danish West Indies, 1803–1848.* Museum Tusculanum Press, University of Copenhagen, Copenhagen.

Jewson, N. D.

1974 Medical Knowledge and the Patronage System in 18th Century England. *Sociology* 8(3): 369–385.

Johnson, Benjamin Heber

2018 *Escaping the Dark, Gray City: Fear and Hope in Progressive-Era Conservation.* Yale University Press, New Haven, Connecticut.

Johnson, Jenell M., Kelly E. Happe, and Marina Levina

2018 Introduction. In *Biocitizenship: The Politics of Bodies, Governance, and Power,* edited by Kelly Happe, Jenell Johnson, and Marina Levina, pp. 1–20. New York University Press, New York.

Johnson, Pamela Jo, Judy Jou, Todd H. Rockwood, and Dawn M. Upchurch

2019 Perceived Benefits of Using Complementary and Alternative Medicine by Race/Ethnicity among Midlife and Older Adults in the United States. *Journal of Aging and Health* 31(8): 1376–1397.

Johnston, Robert D. (editor)

2004 *The Politics of Healing: Histories of Alternative Medicine in Twentieth-Century North America.* Routledge, New York.

Jones, Kari

2019 From Performance to Participation: Fostering a Sense of Shared Heritage Through Archaeology at the Presidio of San Francisco. In *Transforming Heritage Practice in the 21st Century,* edited by John H. Jameson and Sergiu Musteață, pp. 183–196. One World Archaeology. Springer, Cham.

Jones, Olive R.

1981 Essence of Peppermint, a History of the Medicine and Its Bottle. *Historical Archaeology* 15(2): 1–57.

1983 London Mustard Bottles. *Historical Archaeology* 17(1): 69–84.

Joppke, Christian

2007 Transformation of Citizenship: Status, Rights, Identity. *Citizenship Studies* 11(1): 37–48.

Jouanna, Jacques, and Philip van der Eijk

2012 *Greek Medicine from Hippocrates to Galen: Selected Papers.* Studies in Ancient Medicine 40. Brill, Leiden.

Kamat, Vinay R., and Mark Nichter

1998 Pharmacies, Self-Medication and Pharmaceutical Marketing in Bombay, India. *Social Science & Medicine* 47(6): 779–794.

Kell, Katharine T.

1965 Tobacco in Folk Cures in Western Society. *The Journal of American Folklore* 78(308): 99.

Key, Jack D.

1968 U.S. Army Medical Department and Civil War Medicine. *Military Medicine* 133(3): 181–192.

Komara, Zada

2023 Healer's Choice: Gender, Self-Care, and Women's Wellness Products in an Appalachian Coal Town. *International Journal of Historical Archaeology* 27(1): 158–182.

Krieger, Nancy

1992   The Making of Public Health Data: Paradigms, Politics, and Policy. *Journal of Public Health Policy* 13(4): 412.

1999   Embodying Inequality: A Review of Concepts, Measures, and Methods for Studying Health Consequences of Discrimination. *International Journal of Health Services* 29(2): 295–352.

Kuglitsch, Linnea

2023   All the Aids that Nature Can Afford: Horticulture, Healing, and Moral Reform in a Gilded Age Hospital. *International Journal of Historical Archaeology* 27(1): 183–200.

Lamb, Sarah

2019   On Being (Not) Old: Agency, Self-Care, and Life-Course Aspirations in the United States. *Medical Anthropology Quarterly* 33(2): 263–281.

Lans, Aja M.

2022   Investigating Black Women's Mental Health in Progressive Era New York City: A Bioarchaeological Study of Slow Violence and Landscapes of Impunity. *Historical Archaeology* 56(4): 663–680.

Lanska, Douglas

1989   The History of Reflex Hammers. *Neurology* 39(11): 1542–1542.

Larsen, Clark Spencer

2002   Bioarchaeology: The Lives and Lifestyles of Past People. *Journal of Archaeological Research* 10(2): 119–166.

2018   The Bioarchaeology of Health Crisis: Infectious Disease in the Past. *Annual Review of Anthropology* 47(1): 295–313.

Larsen, Clark Spencer, Mark C. Griffin, Dale L. Hutchinson, Vivian E. Noble, Lynette Norr, Robert F. Pastor, Christopher B. Ruff, et al.

2001   Frontiers of Contact: Bioarchaeology of Spanish Florida. *Journal of World Prehistory* 15(1): 69–123.

Larsen, Eric L.

1994   A Boardinghouse Madonna—Beyond the Aesthetics of a Portrait Created Through Medicine Bottles. *Historical Archaeology* 28(4): 68–79.

Lasco, Gideon

2020   Medical Populism and the COVID-19 Pandemic. *Global Public Health* 15(10): 1417–1429.

Lawlor, Clark, and Akihito Suzuki

2000   The Disease of the Self: Representing Consumption, 1700–1830. *Bulletin of the History of Medicine* 74(3): 458–494.

Lee, Lori A.

2017   Health Consumerism Among Enslaved Virginians. In *Material Worlds: Archaeology, Consumption, and the Road to Modernity,* edited by Barbara J. Heath, Eleanor E. Breen, and Lori A. Lee, pp. 141–161. Routledge Studies in Archaeology 26. Routledge/Taylor & Francis Group, London and New York.

Legan, Marshall Scott

1971 Hydropathy in America: A Nineteenth Century Panacea. *Bulletin of the History of Medicine* 45(3): 267–280.

Lightfoot, Kent G.

1995 Culture Contact Studies: Redefining the Relationship Between Prehistoric and Historical Archaeology. *American Antiquity* 60(2): 199–217.

Lightfoot, Kent G., Lee M. Panich, Tsim D. Schneider, and Sara L. Gonzalez

2013 European Colonialism and the Anthropocene: A View from the Pacific Coast of North America. *Anthropocene* 4: 101–115.

Linn, Meredith B.

2008 From Typhus to Tuberculosis and Fractures in Between: A Visceral Historical Archaeology of Irish Immigrant Life in New York City, 1845–1870. PhD dissertation, Department of Anthropology, Columbia University, New York.

2010 Elixir of Emigration: Soda Water and the Making of Irish Americans in Nineteenth-Century New York City. *Historical Archaeology* 44(4): 69–109.

Lippert, Frank

2013 An Introduction to Toothpaste—Its Purpose, History and Ingredients. In *Monographs in Oral Science,* edited by C. van Loveren, pp. 1–14. S. Karger, Basel.

Liu, Danting, Margaret Schmitt, Azure Nowara, Cathryn Magno, Rebecca Ortiz, and Marni Sommer

2021 The Evolving Landscape of Menstrual Product Advertisements in the United States: 2008–2018. *Health Care for Women International:* 1–28.

London Standard

1831 Advertisement, 7 June: 1.

Loren, Diana DiPaolo

2013 Considering Mimicry and Hybridity in Early Colonial New England: Health, Sin and the Body "Behung with Beades." In *Archaeology and Cultural Mixture: Creolization, Hybridity and Mestizaje,* edited by W. Paul van Pelt, pp. 151–168. Cambridge University Press, Cambridge.

2015 Dress, Faith, and Medicine: Caring for the Body in Eighteenth-Century Spanish Texas. In *Archaeology of Culture Contact and Colonialism in Spanish and Portuguese America,* edited by Pedro Paulo A. Funari and Maria Ximena Senatore, pp. 143–153. Springer, Cham.

2016 Bodily Protection: Dress, Health, and Anxiety in Colonial New England. In *The Archaeology of Anxiety,* edited by Jeffrey Fleisher and Neil Norman, pp. 141–156. Springer, New York.

Lovell, W. George

1992 "Heavy Shadows and Black Night": Disease and Depopulation in Colonial Spanish America. *Annals of the Association of American Geographers* 82(3): 426–443.

Lupton, Deborah

1993 Risk as Moral Danger: The Social and Political Functions of Risk Discourse in Public Health. *International Journal of Health Services* 23(3): 425–435.

1997 *The Imperative of Health: Public Health and the Regulated Body.* Sage, Thousand Oaks, California.

2012 *Medicine as Culture: Illness, Disease, and the Body.* 3rd ed. Sage, Los Angeles.

Lyles, Alan

2002 Direct Marketing of Pharmaceuticals to Consumers. *Annual Review of Public Health* 23(1): 73–91.

Macey, David

2009 Rethinking Biopolitics, Race and Power in the Wake of Foucault. *Theory, Culture & Society* 26(6): 186–205.

Majewski, Teresita, and Michael Brian Schiffer

2009 Beyond Consumption: Toward an Archaeology of Consumerism. In *International Handbook of Historical Archaeology,* edited by David Gaimster and Teresita Majewski, pp. 191–207. Springer, New York.

Maniery, Mary L.

2002 Health, Sanitation, and Diet in a Twentieth-Century Dam Construction Camp: A View from Butt Valley, California. *Historical Archaeology* 36(3): 69–84.

Mant, Madeleine, Carlina Cova, and Megan B. Brickley

2021 Intersectionality and Trauma Analysis in Bioarchaeology. *American Journal of Physical Anthropology* 174(4): 583–594.

Mant, Madeleine L., and Alyson Holland

2019 *Bioarchaeology of Marginalized People.* Academic Press, London.

Marcellus, Jane

2008 Nervous Women and Noble Savages: The Romanticized "Other" in Nineteenth-Century Patent Medicine Advertising. *Journal of Popular Culture* 41(5): 784–808.

Marmot, Michael

2005 Social Determinants of Health Inequalities. *The Lancet* 365(9464): 1099–1104.

Marshall, James D.

1997 Michel Foucault: Problematising the Individual and Constituting "the" Self. *Educational Philosophy and Theory* 29(1): 32–49.

Martin, Debra L., Ryan P. Harrod, and Ventura R. Pérez

2013 *Bioarchaeology: An Integrated Approach to Working with Human Remains.* Manuals in Archaeological Method, Theory and Technique. Springer, New York.

Mason, Paul H., Anupom Roy, Jayden Spillane, and Puneet Singh

2016 Social, Historical, and Cultural Dimensions of Tuberculosis. *Journal of Biosocial Science* 48(2): 206–232.

Matthew, Dayna Bowen

2018 *Just Medicine: A Cure for Racial Inequality in American Health Care.* New York University Press, New York.

Mbembe, Achille

2008 Necropolitics. In *Foucault in an Age of Terror,* edited by Stephen Morton and Stephen Bygrave, pp. 152–182. Palgrave Macmillan UK, London.

McClean, Stuart, and Mary Mitchell

2018   "You Feel It in Your Body": Narratives of Embodied Well-Being and Control Among Women Who Use Complementary and Alternative Medicine During Pregnancy. *Societies* 8(2): 30.

McClintock, Anne

2005   Soft-Soaping Empire: Commodity Racism and Imperial Advertising. In *The Body: A Reader,* edited by Mariam Fraser and Monica Greco, pp. 267–270. Routledge, New York.

2013   *Imperial Leather: Race, Gender, and Sexuality in the Colonial Contest.* Taylor & Francis, Hoboken.

McFarland, Bentson, Douglas Bigelow, Brigid Zani, Jason Newsom, and Mark Kaplan

2002   Complementary and Alternative Medicine Use in Canada and the United States. *American Journal of Public Health* 92(10): 1616–1618.

McGillivray, David

2005   Fitter, Happier, More Productive: Governing Working Bodies through Wellness. *Culture and Organization* 11(2): 125–138.

McLeod, Kari S.

2000   Our Sense of Snow: The Myth of John Snow in Medical Geography. *Social Science & Medicine* 50(7–8): 923–935.

Miller, Holly, and Naomi Sykes

2016   Zootherapy in Archaeology: The Case of the Fallow Deer (*Dama dama dama*). *Journal of Ethnobiology* 36(2): 257–276.

Milner, George R., and Jesper L. Boldsen

2017   Life Not Death: Epidemiology from Skeletons. *International Journal of Paleopathology* 17: 26–39.

Mishra, Vaibhav, Golnoush Seyedzenouzi, Ahmad Almohtadi, Tasnim Chowdhury, Arwa Khashkhusha, Ariana Axiaq, Wing Yan Elizabeth Wong, and Amer Harky

2021   Health Inequalities During COVID-19 and Their Effects on Morbidity and Mortality. *Journal of Healthcare Leadership* 13: 19–26.

Mitchell, Peter

2003   The Archaeological Study of Epidemic and Infectious Disease. *World Archaeology* 35(2): 171–179.

Mol, Annemarie

2008   *The Logic of Care.* Routledge, New York.

Mol, Annemarie, Ingunn Moser, and Jeannette Pols (editors)

2010   *Care in Practice: On Tinkering in Clinics, Homes and Farms.* Transcript Verlag, Bielefeld.

Montesi, Laura

2020   "If I Don't Take Care of Myself, Who Will?" Self-Caring Subjects in Oaxaca's Mutual-Aid Groups. *Anthropology & Medicine* 27(4): 380–394.

Morantz, Regina Markell

1977   Making Women Modern: Middle Class Women and Health Reform in 19th Century America. *Journal of Social History* 10(4): 490–507.

Morantz-Sanchez, Regina

2005 *Sympathy and Science: Women Physicians in American Medicine.* The University of North Carolina Press, Charlottesville.

Morton, Ashley

2013 Freedom from Worry: Douching as a Case Study for Historical Archaeological Approaches to Women's Health. MA Thesis, Department of Anthropology, University of Idaho.

Moynihan, R.

2002 Selling Sickness: The Pharmaceutical Industry and Disease Mongering. Commentary: Medicalisation of Risk Factors. *BMJ* 324(7342): 886–891.

Mrozowski, S. A., E. L. Bell, M. C. Beaudry, D. B. Landon, and G. K. Kelso

1989 Living on the Boott: Health and Well Being in a Boardinghouse Population. *World Archaeology* 21(2): 298–319.

Mrozowski, Stephen A., Maria Franklin, and Leslie Hunt

2008 Archaeobotanical Analysis and Interpretations of Enslaved Virginian Plant Use at Rich Neck Plantation (44WB52). *American Antiquity* 73(4): 699–728.

Muller, Jennifer L., Kristen E. Pearlstein, and Carlina de la Cova

2017 Dissection and Documented Skeletal Collections: Embodiments of Legalized Inequality. In *The Bioarchaeology of Dissection and Autopsy in the United States,* edited by Kenneth C. Nystrom, pp. 185–201. Springer, Cham.

Mullins, Paul R.

2011 The Archaeology of Consumption. *Annual Review of Anthropology* 40(1): 133–144.

2012 *The Archaeology of Consumer Culture.* The American Experience in Archaeological Perspective. University Press of Florida, Gainesville.

Murphy, Melissa Scott, Haagen D. Klaus, and Clark Spencer Larsen

2017 *Colonized Bodies, Worlds Transformed: Toward a Global Bioarchaeology of Contact and Colonialism.* University Press of Florida, Gainesville.

Musto, David F.

1999 *The American Disease: Origins of Narcotic Control.* Oxford University Press, New York.

Narasimhan, Padmanesan, James Wood, Chandini Raina MacIntyre, and Dilip Mathai

2013 Risk Factors for Tuberculosis. *Pulmonary Medicine* 2013: 1–11.

National Museum of American History.

n.d. E. Pinaud Eau de Quinine Compound Hair Tonic. National Museum of American History, https://americanhistory.si.edu/collections/search/object/nmah_209778, accessed February 7, 2024.

Nichter, Mark

1996 Pharmaceuticals, Health Commodification, and Social Relations: Ramifications for Primary Health Care. In *Anthropology and International Health,* edited by Mark Nichter and Mimi Nichter, pp. 233–277. Routledge, New York.

Ning, Ana M.

2013 How "Alternative" Is CAM? Rethinking Conventional Dichotomies Between Biomedicine and Complementary/Alternative Medicine. *Health: An Interdis-*

ciplinary Journal for the Social Study of Health, Illness and Medicine 17(2): 135–158.

Novak, Shannon A.

2017 Partible Persons or Persons Apart: Postmortem Interventions at the Spring Street Presbyterian Church, Manhattan. In *The Bioarchaeology of Dissection and Autopsy in the United States,* edited by Kenneth C. Nystrom, pp. 87–111. Bioarchaeology and Social Theory. Springer, Cham.

Nye, Robert A.

2003 The Evolution of the Concept of Medicalization in the Late Twentieth Century. *Journal of the History of the Behavioral Sciences* 39(2): 115–129.

Nystrom, Kenneth C.

2014 The Bioarchaeology of Structural Violence and Dissection in the 19th-Century United States. *American Anthropologist* 116(4): 765–779.

Nystrom, Kenneth C. (editor)

2017 *The Bioarchaeology of Dissection and Autopsy in the United States.* Bioarchaeology and Social Theory. Springer, Cham.

Nystrom, Kenneth C., Joyce Sirianni, Rosanne Higgins, Douglas Perrelli, and Jennifer L. Liber Raines

2017 Structural Inequality and Postmortem Examination at the Erie County Poorhouse. In *The Bioarchaeology of Dissection and Autopsy in the United States,* edited by Kenneth C. Nystrom, pp. 279–300. Springer, Cham.

Ockenhouse, Christian F., Alan Magill, Dale Smith, and Wil Milhous

2005 History of U.S. Military Contributions to the Study of Malaria. *Military Medicine* 170(4S): 12–16.

Oldstone-Moore, Christopher

2015 *Of Beards and Men: The Revealing History of Facial Hair.* University of Chicago Press, Chicago, Illinois.

Ong, Aihwa, Virginia R. Dominguez, Jonathan Friedman, Nina Glick Schiller, Verena Stolcke, and Hu Ying

1996 Cultural Citizenship as Subject-Making: Immigrants Negotiate Racial and Cultural Boundaries in the United States [and Comments and Reply]. *Current Anthropology* 37(5): 737–762.

Orser, Charles E.

1990 Archaeological Approaches to New World Plantation Slavery. *Archaeological Method and Theory* 2: 111–154.

1994 Consumption, Consumerism, and Things from the Earth. *Historical Methods: A Journal of Quantitative and Interdisciplinary History* 27(2): 61–70.

1996 *A Historical Archaeology of the Modern World.* Contributions to Global Historical Archaeology. Springer, Boston, Massachusetts.

2010 Twenty-First-Century Historical Archaeology. *Journal of Archaeological Research* 18(2): 111–150.

2016 *Historical Archaeology.* Routledge, New York.

Ott, Katherine

1996   *Fevered Lives: Tuberculosis in American Culture since 1870.* Harvard University Press, Cambridge, Massachusetts.

Pagel, Walter

1955   Humoral Pathology: A Lingering Anachronism in the History of Tuberculosis. *Bulletin of the History of Medicine* 29(4): 299–308.

Panich, Lee M.

2013   Archaeologies of Persistence: Reconsidering the Legacies of Colonialism in Native North America. *American Antiquity* 78(1): 105–122.

Panich, Lee M., Helga Afaghani, and Nicole Mathwich

2014   Assessing the Diversity of Mission Populations through the Comparison of Native American Residences at Mission Santa Clara de Asís. *International Journal of Historical Archaeology* 18(3): 467–488.

Panich, Lee M., and Tsim D. Schneider

2015   Expanding Mission Archaeology: A Landscape Approach to Indigenous Autonomy in Colonial California. *Journal of Anthropological Archaeology* 40: 48–58.

Panter-Brick, Catherine, and Mark Eggerman

2018   The Field of Medical Anthropology in Social Science & Medicine. *Social Science & Medicine* 196: 233–239.

Park, Shelley

1996   From Sanitation to Liberation: The Modern and Postmodern Marketing of Menstrual Products. *Journal of Popular Culture* 30(2): 149–168.

Patel, J. A., F.B.H. Nielsen, A. A. Badiani, S. Assi, V. A. Unadkat, B. Patel, R. Ravindrane, and H. Wardle

2020   Poverty, Inequality and Covid-19: The Forgotten Vulnerable. *Public Health* 183: 110–111.

Pearce, N.

1996   Traditional Epidemiology, Modern Epidemiology, and Public Health. *American Journal of Public Health* 86(5): 678–683.

Petersen, Alan, and Deborah Lupton

1996   *The New Public Health: Health and Self in the Age of Risk.* Sage, Thousand Oaks, California.

Peterson, Jon A.

1979   The Impact of Sanitary Reform upon American Urban Planning, 1840–1890. *Journal of Social History* 13(1): 83–103.

Petit, Jeanne

2021   "See Him Through": Masculinity and the War Work of the Knights of Columbus, 1917–1918. *American Catholic Studies* 132(2): 22–28.

Petryna, Adriana

2004   Biological Citizenship: The Science and Politics of Chernobyl-Exposed Populations. *Osiris* 19(1): 250–265.

Picard, Alyssa

2009 *Making the American Mouth: Dentists and Public Health in the Twentieth Century.* Rutgers University Press, New Brunswick, New Jersey.

Porter, Dorothy

2005 *Health, Civilization, and the State: A History of Public Health from Ancient to Modern Times.* Routledge, New York.

Porter, Roy

2003 *Patients and Practitioners: Lay Perceptions of Medicine in Pre-industrial Society.* Cambridge University Press, Cambridge.

Portman, Tarrell A. A., and Michael T. Garrett

2006 Native American Healing Traditions. *International Journal of Disability, Development and Education* 53(4): 453–469.

Powell, Lindsay, William Southwell-Wright, and Rebecca Gowland (editors)

2017 *Care in the Past: Archaeological and Interdisciplinary Perspectives.* Oxbow, Philadelphia, Pennsylvania.

Procter & Gamble

2023 History of Gillette. Gillette, https://gillette.com/en-us/about/our-story, accessed February 6, 2024.

Psota, Sunshine

2011 The Archaeology of Mental Illness from the Afflicted and Caretaker Perspective: A Northern California Family's Odyssey. *Historical Archaeology* 45(4): 20–38.

Rabinow, Paul

2005 Artificiality and Enlightenment: From Sociobiology to Biosociality. In *Anthropologies of Modernity,* edited by Jonathan Xavier Inda, pp. 179–193. Blackwell, Oxford.

Ramsey, Matthew

2002 *Professional and Popular Medicine in France, 1770–1830: The Social World of Medical Practice.* Cambridge University Press, Cambridge.

Reifschneider, Meredith

2018 Enslavement and Institutionalized Care: The Politics of Health in Nineteenth-Century St Croix, Danish West Indies. *World Archaeology* 50(3): 494–511.

2019 Danish Colonial Healthcare Policy, St. Croix, Virgin Islands. *Itinerario* 43(02): 305–326.

Reifschneider, Meredith, and Dana N. Bardolph

2020 An Archaeobotanical Approach to Well-Being: Enslaved Plant Use at Estate Cane Garden, 19th Century St. Croix. *Journal of Field Archaeology* 45(7): 512–526.

Reilly, Kimberley A.

2014 "A Perilous Venture for Democracy": Soldiers, Sexual Purity, and American Citizenship in the First World War. *The Journal of the Gilded Age and Progressive Era* 13(2): 223–255.

References

Reinhard, Karl

1992   Parasitology as an Interpretive Tool in Archaeology. *American Antiquity* 57(2): 231–245.

2017   Reestablishing Rigor in Archaeological Parasitology. *International Journal of Paleopathology* 19: 124–134.

Reinhard, K. J., L. F. Ferreira, F. Bouchet, L. Sianto, J.M.F. Dutra, A. Iniguez, D. Leles, et al.

2013   Food, Parasites, and Epidemiological Transitions: A Broad Perspective. *International Journal of Paleopathology* 3(3): 150–157.

Richardson, Ruth

2001   *Death, Dissection, and the Destitute.* 2nd ed. University of Chicago Press, Chicago, Illinois.

Riede, Felix

2017   Past-Forwarding Ancient Calamities. Pathways for Making Archaeology Relevant in Disaster Risk Reduction Research. *Humanities* 6(4): 79.

Risse, Guenter B.

2016   *Driven by Fear: Epidemics and Isolation in San Francisco's House of Pestilence.* University of Illinois Press, Urbana.

Roberts, Charlotte

2020   Fashionable but Debilitating Diseases: Tuberculosis Past and Present. In *Purposeful Pain: The Bioarchaeology of Intentional Suffering,* edited by Susan Guise Sheridan and Lesley A. Gregoricka, pp. 21–38. Springer, Cham.

Roberts, Charlotte A., and Jane E. Buikstra

2003   *The Bioarchaeology of Tuberculosis: A Global View on a Reemerging Disease.* University Press of Florida, Gainesville.

Roberts, Charlotte, and Keith Manchester

2010   *The Archaeology of Disease.* History Press, Stroud.

Roberts, Dorothy E.

2017   *Killing the Black Body: Race, Reproduction, and the Meaning of Liberty.* Vintage Books, New York.

Rose, Nikolas S.

1999   *Powers of Freedom: Reframing Political Thought.* Cambridge University Press, Cambridge.

Rose, Nikolas, and Carlos Novas

2005   Biological Citizenship. In *Global Assemblages: Technology, Politics, and Ethics as Anthropological Problems,* edited by Aihwa Ong and Stephen Collier, pp. 439–463. Blackwell, New York.

Rosen, George

1953   Cameralism and the Concept of Medical Police. *Bulletin of the History of Medicine* 27(1): 21–42.

2015   *A History of Public Health.* Rev. expand. ed. Johns Hopkins University Press, Baltimore, Maryland.

Rosenberg, Charles E.

1977   The Therapeutic Revolution: Medicine, Meaning, and Social Change in Nineteenth-Century America. *Perspectives in Biology and Medicine* 20(4): 485–506.

Rosenberg, Charles E. (editor)

2003   *Right Living: An Anglo-American Tradition of Self-Help Medicine and Hygiene.* Johns Hopkins University Press, Baltimore, Maryland.

Rothstein, William G.

1987   *American Medical Schools and the Practice of Medicine: A History.* Oxford University Press, Oxford.

Rotman, Deborah L.

2010   The Fighting Irish: Historical Archaeology of Nineteenth-Century Catholic Immigrant Experiences in South Bend, Indiana. *Historical Archaeology* 44(2): 113–131.

Rydland, Håvard Thorsen, Joseph Friedman, Silvia Stringhini, Bruce G. Link, and Terje Andreas Eikemo

2022   The Radically Unequal Distribution of Covid-19 Vaccinations: A Predictable Yet Avoidable Symptom of the Fundamental Causes of Inequality. *Humanities and Social Sciences Communications* 9(1): 61.

Ryzewski, Krysta

2007   Epidemic of Medicine: An Archaeological Dose of Popular Culture. In *Contemporary and Historical Archaeology in Theory: Papers from the 2003 and 2004 CHAT Conferences,* pp. 15–22. Studies in Contemporary and Historical Archaeology 4. Archaeopress, Oxford.

Saltonstall, Robin

1993   Healthy Bodies, Social Bodies: Men's and Women's Concepts and Practices of Health in Everyday Life. *Social Science & Medicine* 36(1): 7–14.

Sanabria, Emilia

2015   Circulating Ignorance: Complexity and Agnogenesis in the Obesity "Epidemic." *Cultural Anthropology* 31(1): 131–158.

Savitt, Todd L.

1982   The Use of Blacks for Medical Experimentation and Demonstration in the Old South. *The Journal of Southern History* 48(3): 331.

Savitz, David A.

2003   *Interpreting Epidemiologic Evidence: Strategies for Study Design and Analysis.* Oxford University Press, Oxford.

Scheidel, Walter

2018   *The Great Leveler: Violence and the History of Inequality from the Stone Age to the Twenty-First Century.* Princeton University Press, Princeton, New Jersey.

Scheper-Hughes, Nancy, and Margaret M. Lock

1987   The Mindful Body: A Prolegomenon to Future Work in Medical Anthropology. *Medical Anthropology Quarterly* 1(1): 6–41.

Schiffer, Michael B.

1992 *Technological Perspectives on Behavioral Change.* Culture and Technology. University of Arizona Press, Tucson.

Schwartz, Lisa M., and Steven Woloshin

2019 Medical Marketing in the United States, 1997–2016. *JAMA* 321(1): 80.

Scott, Alyssa Rose

2023 Archaeology, Disability, Healthcare, and the Weimar Joint Sanatorium for Tuberculosis. *International Journal of Historical Archaeology* 27(1): 201–219.

Scott, Douglas D., and Andrew P. McFeaters

2011 The Archaeology of Historic Battlefields: A History and Theoretical Development in Conflict Archaeology. *Journal of Archaeological Research* 19(1): 103–132.

Scott, James

2008 *Weapons of the Weak.* Yale University Press, New Haven, Connecticut.

Segal, Judy Z.

2020 The Empowered Patient on a Historical-Rhetorical Model: 19th-Century Patent-Medicine Ads and the 21st-Century Health Subject. *Health: An Interdisciplinary Journal for the Social Study of Health, Illness and Medicine* 24(5): 572–588.

Shackel, Paul A.

1993 *Personal Discipline and Material Culture: An Archaeology of Annapolis, Maryland, 1695–1870.* University of Tennessee Press, Knoxville.

Shah, Nayan

2001 *Contagious Divides: Epidemics and Race in San Francisco's Chinatown.* American Crossroads. University of California Press, Berkeley.

Shaw, Julia, and Naomi Sykes

2018 New Directions in the Archaeology of Medicine: Deep-Time Approaches to Human-Animal-Environmental Care. *World Archaeology* 50(3): 365–383.

Sheridan, Susan Guise, and Lesley A. Gregoricka (editors)

2020 *Purposeful Pain: The Bioarchaeology of Intentional Suffering.* Bioarchaeology and Social Theory. Springer, Cham.

Shortt, S. E. D.

1983 Physicians, Science, and Status: Issues in the Professionalization of Anglo-American Medicine in the Nineteenth Century. *Medical History* 27(1): 51–68.

Shryock, Richard Harrison

1936 *The Development of Modern Medicine: An Interpretation of the Social and Scientific Factors Involved.* University of Pennsylvania Press, Philadelphia.

Shuler, Kristina

2011 Life and Death on a Barbadian Sugar Plantation: Historic and Bioarchaeological Views of Infection and Mortality at Newton Plantation. *International Journal of Osteoarchaeology* 21(1): 66–81.

Shultz, Suzanne M.

2005 *Body Snatching: The Robbing of Graves for the Education of Physicians in Early Nineteenth Century America.* McFarland, Jefferson, North Carolina.

Sikand, Anju, and Marilyn Laken

1998   Pediatricians' Experience with and Attitudes toward Complementary/Alternative Medicine. *Archives of Pediatrics & Adolescent Medicine* 152(11): 1059–1064.

Silliman, Stephen W.

2005   "Culture Contact or Colonialism? Challenges in the Archaeology of Native North America." *American Antiquity* 70(1): 55–74.

Simmons, James Stephens

1943   The Preventive Medicine Program of the United States Army. *American Journal of Public Health* 33: 931–940.

Singh, Gopal, Gem Daus, Michelle Allender, Christine Ramey, Elijah Martin, Chrisp Perry, Andrew Reyes, and Ivy Vedamuthu

2017   Social Determinants of Health in the United States: Addressing Major Health Inequality Trends for the Nation, 1935–2016. *International Journal of MCH and AIDS* 6(2): 139–164.

Singleton, Theresa A.

1995   The Archaeology of Slavery in North America. *Annual Review of Anthropology* 24(1): 119–140.

Slominski, Kristy L.

2021   Moral Education about Sex in the YMCA and Military. In *Teaching Moral Sex: A History of Religion and Sex Education in the United States,* edited by Kristy Slominski, pp. 67–122. Oxford University Press, Oxford.

Smith, Monica L.

2007   Inconspicuous Consumption: Non-display Goods and Identity Formation. *Journal of Archaeological Method and Theory* 14(4): 412–438.

Smith, Virginia

2008   *Clean: A History of Personal Hygiene and Purity.* Oxford University Press, Oxford.

Smith-Morris, Carolyn

2018   Care as Virtue, Care as Critical Frame: A Discussion of Four Recent Ethnographies. *Medical Anthropology* 37(5): 426–432.

Soja, Edward W.

1996   *Thirdspace: Journeys to Los Angeles and Other Real-and-Imagined Places.* Blackwell, Cambridge, Massachusetts.

Sokolov, Barbara Berglund, and John Bertland

2020   Letterman General Hospital during World War I. *California History* 97(3): 86–121.

Sontag, Susan

2001   *Illness as Metaphor and AIDS and Its Metaphors.* Picador, New York.

Spencer-Wood, Suzanne M.

2001   Introduction and Historical Context to the Archaeology of Seventeenth and Eighteenth Century Almshouses. *International Journal of Historical Archaeology* 5(2): 115–122.

Spencer-Wood, Suzanne M., and Sherene Baugher

2001 Introduction and Historical Context for the Archaeology of Institutions of Reform. Part I: Asylums. *International Journal of Historical Archaeology* 5(1): 3–17.

Spencer-Wood, Suzanne M., and Scott D. Heberling

1987 Consumer Choices in White Ceramics. In *Consumer Choice in Historical Archaeology,* edited by Suzanne M. Spencer-Wood, pp. 55–84. Springer, Boston, Massachusetts.

Stahnisch, Frank W., and Marja Verhoef

2012 The Flexner Report of 1910 and Its Impact on Complementary and Alternative Medicine and Psychiatry in North America in the 20th Century. *Evidence-Based Complementary and Alternative Medicine* 2012: 647896.

Star, Susan Leigh, and James R. Griesemer

1989 Institutional Ecology, "Translations" and Boundary Objects: Amateurs and Professionals in Berkeley's Museum of Vertebrate Zoology, 1907–39. *Social Studies of Science* 19(3): 387–420.

Starbuck, David R.

2011 *The Archaeology of Forts and Battlefields.* University Press of Florida, Gainesville.

Starr, Paul

2009 Professionalization and Public Health: Historical Legacies, Continuing Dilemmas. *Journal of Public Health Management and Practice* 15(Supplement): S26–S30.

2017 *The Social Transformation of American Medicine.* 2nd ed. Basic Books, New York.

Steele, Caroline

2008 Archaeology and the Forensic Investigation of Recent Mass Graves: Ethical Issues for a New Practice of Archaeology. *Archaeologies* 4(3): 414–428.

Steinecke, Ann, and Charles Terrell

2010 Progress for Whose Future? The Impact of the Flexner Report on Medical Education for Racial and Ethnic Minority Physicians in the United States. *Academic Medicine* 85(2): 236–245.

Stojanowski, Christopher M.

2005 The Bioarchaeology of Identity in Spanish Colonial Florida: Social and Evolutionary Transformation before, during, and after Demographic Collapse. *American Anthropologist* 107(3): 417–431.

Storey, Nicholas

2011 *A Short Guide for Men about Town: A Short Miscellany, Including Some Unusual Titbits and Tips on Grooming, Accessories and Fine Living.* Barnsley, South Yorkshire.

Storm, Erica M.

2018 Roy Porter Student Prize Essay, Gilding the Pill: The Sensuous Consumption of Patent Medicines, 1815–1841. *Social History of Medicine* 31(1): 41–60.

Stottman, M. Jay
2000   Out of Sight, Out of Mind: Privy Architecture and the Perception of Sanitation. *Historical Archaeology* 34(1): 39–61.

Stradling, David (editor)
2004   *Conservation in the Progressive Era: Classic Texts.* University of Washington Press, Seattle.

Stratton, Samuel J.
2020   COVID-19: Not a Simple Public Health Emergency. *Prehospital and Disaster Medicine* 35(2): 119.

Street, John
1917   The Patent Medicine Situation. *American Journal of Public Health* 7(12): 1037–1042.

SturtzSreetharan, Cindi L., Sarah Trainer, Amber Wutich, and Alexandra A. Brewis
2018   Moral Biocitizenship: Discursively Managing Food and the Body after Bariatric Surgery. *Journal of Linguistic Anthropology* 28(2): 221–240.

Sullivan, Louis W., and Ilana Suez Mittman
2010   The State of Diversity in the Health Professions a Century after Flexner: *Academic Medicine* 85(2): 246–253.

Surface-Evans, Sarah
2023   Exploring Well-Being at Three Great Lakes Lighthouses. *International Journal of Historical Archaeology* 27(1): 117–142.

Sutherland, Patsy, Roy Moodley, and Barry Chevannes (editors)
2013   *Caribbean Healing Traditions.* Routledge, New York.

Sutton, Mary-Jean
2003   Re-Examining Total Institutions: A Case Study from Queensland. *Archaeology in Oceania* 38(2): 78–88.

Syme, S. Leonard
2004   Social Determinants of Health: The Community as an Empowered Partner. *Preventing Chronic Disease* 1(1): A02.

Talevi, Alan
2010   The New Patient and Responsible Self-Medication Practices: A Critical Review. *Current Drug Safety* 5(4): 342–353.

Tarlow, Sarah
2012   The Archaeology of Emotion and Affect. *Annual Review of Anthropology* 41(1): 169–185.

Taylor, Jamila K.
2020   Structural Racism and Maternal Health among Black Women. *Journal of Law, Medicine & Ethics* 48(3): 506–517.

Taylor, Robert Joseph, Linda M. Chatters, and Jeffrey S. Levin
2004   *Religion in the Lives of African Americans: Social, Psychological, and Health Perspectives.* Sage, Thousand Oaks, California.

Taylor, Robert Joseph, Christopher G. Ellison, Linda M. Chatters, Jeffrey S. Levin, and Karen D. Lincoln

2000   Mental Health Services in Faith Communities: The Role of Clergy in Black Churches. *Social Work* 45(1): 73–87.

Temin, Peter

1980   Regulation and the Choice of Prescription Drugs. *The American Economic Review* 70(2): 301–305.

Thompson, Erwin

1997   *Defender of the Gate: The Presidio of San Francisco: A History from 1846 to 1995.* U.S. Department of the Interior, National Park Service, Denver Service Center, Denver, Colorado.

Thompson, Kevin

2003   Forms of Resistance: Foucault on Tactical Reversal and Self-Formation. *Continental Philosophy Review* 36(2): 113–138.

Thorne, Sally, Barbara Paterson, Cynthia Russell, and Annette Schultz

2002   Complementary/Alternative Medicine in Chronic Illness as Informed Self-Care Decision Making. *International Journal of Nursing Studies* 39(7): 671–683.

Tilley, Lorna, and A. Schrenck (editors)

2017   *New Developments in the Bioarchaeology of Care.* Springer, New York.

The Times

1840   Advertisement, 7 November.

Tomes, Nancy

2006   Patients or Health Care Consumers? Why the History of Contested Terms Matters. In *History and Health Policy in the United States: Putting the Past Back In,* edited by Rosemary Stevens, Charles E. Rosenberg, and Lawton R. Burns, pp. 83–110. Critical Issues in Health and Medicine. Rutgers University Press, New Brunswick, New Jersey.

2007   Patient Empowerment and the Dilemmas of Late-Modern Medicalisation. *The Lancet* 369(9562): 698–700.

2016   *Remaking the American Patient: How Madison Avenue and Modern Medicine Turned Patients into Consumers.* Studies in Social Medicine. University of North Carolina Press, Chapel Hill.

2020   Patients or Health-Care Consumers? Why the History of Contested Terms Matters. In *History and Health Policy in the United States,* edited by Rosemary A. Stevens, Charles E. Rosenberg, and Lawton R. Burns, pp. 83–110. Rutgers University Press, New York.

2021   "Not Just for Doctors Anymore": How the Merck Manual Became a Consumer Health "Bible." *Bulletin of the History of Medicine* 95(1): 1–23.

Torbenson, Michael, Robert H. Kelly, Jonathon Erlen, Lorna Cropcho, Michael Moraca, Bonnie Beiler, K.N. Rao, and Mohamed Virji

2000   Lash's: A Bitter Medicine: Biochemical Analysis of an Historical Proprietary Medicine. *Historical Archaeology* 34(2): 56–64.

Trombold, John M.

2011   Gangrene Therapy and Antisepsis before Lister: The Civil War Contributions of Middleton Goldsmith of Louisville. *The American Surgeon* 77(9): 1138–1143.

Tung, Tiffiny A.

2021   Making and Marking Maleness and Valorizing Violence: A Bioarchaeological Analysis of Embodiment in the Andean Past. *Current Anthropology* 62(S23): S125–S144.

Tutorow, Norman E.

1996   A Tale of Two Hospitals: U.S. Marine Hospital No. 19 and the U.S. Public Health Service Hospital on the Presidio of San Francisco. *California History* 75(2): 154–169.

United States Food and Drug Administration

1920   *Notices of Judgment Under the Food and Drugs Act Issue 7001, Part 8000.* U.S. Government Printing Office, Washington, DC.

Vallgårda, Signild

1995   The History of Medicine in Denmark. *Social History of Medicine* 8(1): 117–123.

Van Buren, Mary

2010   The Archaeological Study of Spanish Colonialism in the Americas. *Journal of Archaeological Research* 18(2): 151–201.

van Dorn, Aaron, Rebecca E. Cooney, and Miriam L. Sabin

2020   COVID-19 Exacerbating Inequalities in the US. *The Lancet* 395(10232): 1243–1244.

van der Geest, Sjaak, Susan Reynolds Whyte, and Anita Hardon

1996   The Anthropology of Pharmaceuticals: A Biographical Approach. *Annual Review of Anthropology* 25(1): 153–178.

Vanderwarker, Amber M., and Bill Stanyard

2009   Bearsfoot and Deer Legs: Archaeobotanical and Zooarchaeological Evidence of a Special-Purpose Encampment at the Sandy Site, Roanoke, Virginia. *Journal of Ethnobiology* 29(1): 129–148.

Vaughn, Megan

1991   *Curing Their Ills: Colonial Power and African Illness.* Cambridge University Press, Cambridge.

Veit, Richard

1996   "A Ray of Sunshine in the Sickroom": Archaeological Insights into Late 19th- and Early 20th-Century Medicine and Anesthesia. *Northeast Historical Archaeology* 25(1): 33–50.

Verstraete, Emma

2023   Soothing the Self: Medicine Advertisement and the Cult of Domesticity in Nineteenth-Century Springfield, Illinois. *International Journal of Historical Archaeology* 27(1): 143–157.

Voeks, Robert

1993   African Medicine and Magic in the Americas. *Geographical Review* 83(1): 66.

Vogel, Virgil J.

1990   *American Indian Medicine.* University of Oklahoma Press, Norman.

von Wandruszka, Ray, and Mark Warner

2018   A Practical Approach to the Chemical Analysis of Historical Materials. *Historical Archaeology* 52(4): 741–752.

Voss, Barbara L.

2018   The Archaeology of Precarious Lives: Chinese Railroad Workers in Nineteenth-Century North America. *Current Anthropology* 59(3): 287–313.

Voss, Barbara L., Ray von Wandruszka, Alicia Fink, Tara Summer, S. Elizabeth Harman, Anton Shapovalov, Megan S. Kane, Marguerite De Loney, and Nathan Acebo

2015   Stone Drugs and Calamine Lotion: Chemical Analysis of Residue in Nineteenth-Century Glass Bottles, Market Street Chinatown, San Jose, California. *California Archaeology* 7(1): 93–118.

Vuckovic, Nancy, and Mark Nichter

1997   Changing Patterns of Pharmaceutical Practice in the United States. *Social Science & Medicine* 44(9): 1285–1302.

Wagner, Corinna

2015   *Pathological Bodies: Medicine and Political Culture.* University of California Press, Berkeley.

Wald, Priscilla

2020   *Contagious: Cultures, Carriers, and the Outbreak Narrative.* Duke University Press, Durham, North Carolina.

Waldron, Tony

2017   *Palaeoepidemiology: The Measure of Disease in the Human Past.* Routledge, New York.

Walker, Phillip L

2001   A Spanish Borderlands Perspective on La Florida Bioarchaeology. *Bioarchaeology of Spanish Florida: The Impact of Colonialism,* edited by Clark Spencer Larsen, pp. 274–307. University Press of Florida, Gainesville.

Wallis, Patrick, and Brigitte Nerlich

2005   Disease Metaphors in New Epidemics: The UK Media Framing of the 2003 SARS Epidemic. *Social Science & Medicine* 60(11): 2629–2639.

Warner-Smith, Alanna L.

2020   "Views from Somewhere": Mapping Nineteenth-Century Cholera Narratives. *International Journal of Historical Archaeology* 24(4): 877–901.

Washington, Harriet A.

2006   *Medical Apartheid: The Dark History of Medical Experimentation on Black Americans from Colonial Times to the Present.* Doubleday, New York.

Werner, William, and Shannon A. Novak

2010   Archaeologies of Disease and Public Order in Nineteenth-Century New York: The View from Spring and Varick. *Northeast Historical Archaeology* 39(1): 97–119.

White, William A.

2021   Just What the Doctor Ordered: Biochemical Analysis of Historical Medicines from Downtown Tucson, Arizona. *International Journal of Historical Archaeology* 25: 515–543.

Whorton, James C.

2004   *Nature Cures: The History of Alternative Medicine in America*. Oxford University Press, Oxford.

Wilkie, Laurie

1996a   Transforming African American Ethnomedical Traditions: A Case Study from West Feliciana. *Louisiana History: The Journal of the Louisiana Historical Association* 37(4): 457–471.

1996b   Medicinal Teas and Patent Medicines: African-American Women's Consumer Choices and Ethnomedical Traditions at a Louisiana Plantation. *Southeastern Archaeology* 15(2): 119–131.

1997   Secret and Sacred: Contextualizing the Artifacts of African-American Magic and Religion. *Historical Archaeology* 31(4): 81–106.

2000   Magical Passions: Sexuality and African-American Archaeology. In *Archaeologies of Sexuality,* edited by Barbara L. Voss and Robert Schmidt, pp. 129–142. Routledge, London.

2003   *The Archaeology of Mothering: An African-American Midwife's Tale*. Routledge, New York.

2013   Expelling Frogs and Binding Babies: Conception, Gestation and Birth in Nineteenth-Century African-American Midwifery. *World Archaeology* 45(2): 272–284.

2019   At Freedom's Borderland: The Black Regulars and Masculinity at Fort Davis, Texas. *Historical Archaeology* 53(1): 126–137.

2023   Imagining Archaeologies without Ableism. *International Journal of Historical Archaeology* 27(1): 241–266.

Williams, J. Corey, Nientara Anderson, and Dowin Boatright

2021   Beyond Diversity and Inclusion: Reparative Justice in Medical Education. *Academic Psychiatry* 45(1): 84–88.

Winslow, C.-E.A.

1920   The Untilled Fields of Public Health. *Science* 51(1306): 23–33.

Wintermute, Bobby A.

2010   *Public Health and the US Military.* Routledge, London.

Woodbury, Frank, and James Alfred Moss

1918   *Manual for Medical Officers: Being a Guide to the Duties of Army Medical Officers.* George Banta Publishing Company, Menasha, Wisconsin.

Woodhull, Alfred

1890   *Notes on Military Hygiene, for Officers of the Line.* John Wiley & Sons, New York.

Wootton, Jacqueline C.

2005   Classifying and Defining Complementary and Alternative Medicine. *The Journal of Alternative and Complementary Medicine* 11(5): 777–778.

Wurst, LouAnn, and Randall H. McGuire

1999   Immaculate Consumption: A Critique of the "Shop till You Drop" School of Human Behavior. *International Journal of Historical Archaeology* 3(3): 191–199.

Wylie, Alison

2000   "Questions of Evidence, Legitimacy, and the (Dis)Unity of Science." *American Antiquity* 65(2): 227–237.

Xu, H. Daniel, and Rashmita Basu

2020   How the United States Flunked the COVID-19 Test: Some Observations and Several Lessons. *The American Review of Public Administration* 50(6–7): 568–576.

Yamin, Rebecca

1998   Lurid Tales and Homely Stories of New York's Notorious Five Points. *Historical Archaeology* 32(1): 74–85.

Yamin, Rebecca, Pam Crabtree, and Claudia Milne

1997   New York's Mythic Slum. *Archaeology* 50(2): 44–53.

Yamin, Rebecca, and Donna J. Seifert

2023   *The Archaeology of Prostitution and Clandestine Pursuits.* University Press of Florida, Gainesville.

Yates-Doerr, Emily

2012   The Weight of the Self: Care and Compassion in Guatemalan Dietary Choices. *Medical Anthropology Quarterly* 26(1): 136–158.

Young, James Harvey

2015   *The Toadstool Millionaires: A Social History of Patent Medicines in America before Federal Regulation.* Princeton University Press, Princeton, New Jersey.

Yuki, Koichi, Miho Fujiogi, and Sophia Koutsogiannaki

2020   Covid-19 Pathophysiology: A Review. *Clinical Immunology* 215: 108427.

Zebroski, Bob

2016   *A Brief History of Pharmacy: Humanity's Search for Wellness.* Routledge, New York.

Zuckerman, Molly K., and George J. Armelagos

2011   The Origins of Biocultural Dimensions in Bioarchaeology. In *Social Bioarchaeology,* edited by Sabrina Agarwal and Bonnie Glencross, pp. 13–43. Wiley, Hoboken, New Jersey.

Zuckerman, Molly K., Kristin Harper, Ronald Barrett, and George Armelagos

2014   The Evolution of Disease: Anthropological Perspectives on Epidemiologic Transitions. *Global Health Action* 7(1).

Zuckerman, Molly K., Kelly R. Kamnikar, and Sarah A. Mathena

2014   Recovering the "Body Politic": A Relational Ethics of Meaning for Bioarchaeology. *Cambridge Archaeological Journal* 24(3): 513–522.

Zuckerman, Molly K., Anna Grace Tribble, Rita M. Austin, Cassandra M. S. DeGaglia, and Taylor Emery

2022   Biocultural Perspectives on Bioarchaeological and Paleopathological Evidence of Past Pandemics. *American Journal of Biological Anthropology* 182(4): 557–582.

INDEX

Page numbers in *italics* indicate illustrations.

Abortion, 27, 28, 30

Advertising: abortion pills, 28; direct-to-consumer (DTCA), 7, 46–48, 59–60; and health standards, 65; of patent medicines, 52, *52*, 57–58, 59–63, 138; personal hygiene products, 64–65, 136; to professionals, 51; proprietary medicines, 7, 68–69; soda water, 54

African Americans. *See* Black Americans

African Burial Ground Project, New York, 81

African diasporic healing practices, 153

Agnews State Hospital, Stockton, California, 98

Agriculture: plant and animal domestication, 85

Air therapy, 41

Alameda-Stone Cemetery Site, Tucson, Arizona, 58–59

Albany, New York, archaeological sites, 86

Alcohol use, 121, 134, 140–41

Alternative healing systems. *See* CAM (complementary and alternative medicine)

American Medical Association (AMA), 13, 22, 23–24; Council on Medical Education (CME), 24; criticism of patent medicine, 57; Propaganda for Reform Department, 57

Anatomy acts, 20; Anatomy Act of Massachusetts (1831), 21

Anatomy study, 146; anatomical dissection, 18, 20–22

Anesthesia, 20

Animal domestication, 85

Anti-authoritarian approaches, 42

Anti-immigrant discourse, 104–5, 108

Anti-intellectualism, 42

Anza Bezerra Nieto, Juan Bautista, 123

Apothecaries, 33, 52

Archaeology. *See* Bioarchaeology; Historical archaeology; Medical archaeology

Arequipa Sanatorium, 107–9

Arizona Medical Association, 58

Ashe, Thomas, 36

Asylums, xvi, 40–41, 97–98

Author's methodology, 5–12; Presidio artifacts, 127–28

Autopsy, 21–22, 21n2

Baker, Newton, 118

Barnes, Jodi, 63

Bear's-foot (*Polymnia uvedalia*), 36

Beaudry, Mary C., 67

Bedstraw (*Galium* sp.), 36

Beggs Manufacturing Company, 131

Bellevue Hospital, New York, 42

Berlant, Lauren, 153

Berretta, Angelo, 140

Berridge, Virginia, 78

Bioarchaeology: future directions, 149–57; overview and areas of emphasis, 22, 75; public health applications, 80–83, 90. *See also* Historical archaeology; Medical archaeology

Biocitizenship, 9, 76, 78, 104, 110; definitions, 115–16; moral biocitizenship, 116–17; in US Army, 141–42, 144–45

Biocultural approaches to public health, 80–81. *See also* Bioarchaeology

Biomedicine (orthodox medicine): contrasted with CAM, 13–14, 45, 151, 154–55; definitions, 13–14n1; distrust of, 145; prescription vs. patent, 31, 33; professionalization of, xii, 13–14, 16, 147. *See also* Patients; Physicians

196 · Index

Biopolitics, 8, 76, 113
Biopower, 63, 95–96
Black Americans, 146–47; alternative healing systems, 26; Black physicians, 24–25, 32; bodies used for dissection, 21–22; botanical knowledge, 14; community-based health systems, 30–31; freedman hospitals, 31; maternal mortality, 29; midwifery, 29–30; use of patent medicine, 53; women's health, 28–29
Black walnut (*Juglans nigra*), 36
Body-city nexus, 91
Boundaries: "boundary objects," 14; between CAM and biomedicine, 45, 154–55; of diseased spaces, 93
Bromo-Seltzer, 53
Brown, Kathleen M., 122
Brown, Philip, 107–8
Bryant, Lauren, 135
Bucareli, Antonio María, 123
Burdock Blood Bitters, 61
Butt Valley, California, 89

California Labor Camp Sanitation Act, 90
CAM (complementary and alternative medicine), xiii, 11, 13–14n1, 34–38, 145; among diverse communities, 45; contrasted with biomedicine (orthodox medicine), 154–55; current research on, 154–55; current trends, 45, 150–51; delegitimization of, 150–51; marginalized groups, use by, 26
Cancer, 36, 39, 79
Capitalism: capitalist values, 49, 87, 89; consumer capitalism, 50, 71–72; and workplace health, 88
Caribbean plantation hospitals, 149
Carley, Caroline D., 89
Carnegie Foundation, 44
Charitable institutions, 31, 97
Chesebrough petroleum jelly, 130
Childbirth, 27, 28, 29–30; midwifery, 23, 29–30. *See also* Reproductive health care
Children's illnesses, 64
Chinatown, San Francisco, 93–94, 105
Chinese Americans, xiv, 93–94
Chinese medical theories, 55
Chiropractic medicine, 24

Cholera, 18, 32, 85, 93; Caribbean epidemics, 94
Christianity: concepts of physiology, 41; Evangelicalism, 40; Protestant culture and spiritual healing, 39
Cigarettes, 132, 134
Citizenship, 113; American, and moral responsibility, 117; citizenship status and biological existence, 9; definitions, 115; and moral character, 118–23; and personal hygiene, 136. *See also* Biocitizenship
Civil War, 18; public hospitals, 31
Class stratification. *See* Social stratification
Colden, Cadwallader, 35–36
Cold water therapy, 41
Colfax Sanatoria, 107
Colgate toothpaste, 129, 138
Colonialism, 81–82; and concepts of personal hygiene, 122; ecologies of disease, 85–86; European "civilizing" projects, 151
Columbian Exchange, 85–86
Commission on Training Camp Activities (CTCA), 119
Community-based healthcare, xiv–xv, 30–34; marginalized groups, 32–33
"Constitutional pathology," 101–2, 104
Consumerism: consumer behavior and choice, 70–73; consumerism vs. consumption, 49; consumers vs. patients, 69–70; medical consumerism, 46–49
Consumer rights activism, 47
Consumer studies, 49–50
Contraception, 27
Cosmetic advertisements, 63–64
COVID-19 pandemic, xi–xii, 1–3, 74
Covington, Gray, 32
Craddock, Susan, 93–94, 104, 105, 108, 109
Cramp, Arthur, 57
Creese, John L., 72, 83
"Cruel optimism," 153–54
"Cult of domesticity," 61–62
Cutex nail products, 130

Dental care, 137–38
DeWitte, Sharon N., 111
Direct-to-consumer advertising (DTCA), 7, 46–48, 59–60

Disability studies, 4, 107, 148
Disease: social frameworks and metaphor, 99
Dissection, 18, 20–22
"Do it yourself" medicine, 51. *See also* Self-help/self-care
Domesticity and gender roles, 107–9
Domestic medicine, xii-xiii, 25–30, 43. *See also* Self-help/self-care
Donahue, Frank, 20, 41
Drinking water, safety of, 90
Drugs, 131–32, 138–40; advertising, 46; development, 7; federal regulation, 56–59; "off-label" medicine use, 53, 129; OTC drugs, 138–39; recreational drugs, 132, 134. *See also* Patent medicine
Dunnavant, Justin, 30–31

Enslaved persons: Caribbean islands, 37–38; enslaved healers, 68; foodways/medicinal systems, 36–37; Poplar Forest plantation, Virginia, 67–68; slave trade, 37
Environmental pollution, 40
Epidemics: consequences of, 111–12; and European colonization, 85–86. *See also* Infectious disease; Pandemics
Epidemiology, 79
Estate Cane Garden, 38, *38*
Ethnobotanical practices, 14, 35–36
Eugenics, 108
Ex-Lax, 132, 139–140

Farmer, Paul, 110
Feminine hygiene products, 63, 64–65
Finger/Sengstacken household, 98
Fisher, Charles L., 86
Five Points, New York, 32–33, 42, 92, *93*, 110; Courthouse Block, 54–55
Flannery, Michael A., 42
Flexner, Abraham, 24
Flexner Report, 24–25, 44
Food and Drug Administration (FDA), 57
Food/medicine, binary vs. blending, 36–37
Fort Vancouver, Washington, 89
Fosdick, Raymond, 118
Foucault, Michel, 8, 12, 63, 76, 89, 91, 95–96, 97
Fowler, Lydia Folger, 28

Free Young Men's Benevolent Association, 31
Friendly Botanic Society, 43

Galen, 16
Gender roles, 62–63, 107–9. *See also* Women
Germ theory, 92
Gillette razor blades, 130
Ginsburg, Faye, 29
Gleason, Rachel Brooks, 28
Graunt, Edward, 83
Great Western Power (GWP) Company, 90
Greenwich Village, New York, 91–92

Harpers Ferry National Historical Park, West Virginia, 64
Harvard Anatomical Society, 21
Harvard Medical School, 21
Health: individual responsibility, 152; patient choice in health care, 153; perceptions of, 66–67; personal responsibility, 116. *See also* Public health
Health insurance, 70
Health optimization programs, 94–95
Health protection/improvement, 78. *See also* Public health
Health reform movements, 28, 95
Heath, Barbara J., 49
Heffner, Sarah C., 55
Herbal healing practices, 33, 35, 110–11
Heroic medicine, 16–17
"Hidden transcripts," xiii, 6–7
Hippocratic theories, 16, 17, 88
Historical archaeology: background and overview, 3; bottom-up approaches, 154; Foucault's influence, 95–96, 97; health and medicine, 4–5; methodology, 3–4; Native Americans, 81–83; public vs. private space, 156; slavery and colonialism, 81–82; US military spaces, 128–29. *See also* Bioarchaeology; Medical archaeology
Holden Chapel, Harvard, 21
Holistic healing, 34–38. *See also* CAM (complementary and alternative medicine)
Holly seeds (*Ilex vomitoria*), 36
Hollywood Plantation, Arkansas, 29, 43, 63–64, 68–69
Homeopathy, 24, 28, 43

198 · Index

Honey locust (*Gleditsia triacanthos*), 36
Horticultural therapy, 41
Hosek, Lauren, 117
Household medicine, 25–30, 43. *See also* Self-help/self-care
Howson, Jean E., 91–92
Hudson Bay Company, 89
Humoral elements, 16
Hutchinson, Dale L., 82
Hydropathy, 54
Hydrotherapy, 41–42

Immigrants: "Americanization" in US Army, 118; and concepts of personal hygiene, 122; moral judgment of, 152
Indian pokeroot (*Phytolacca decandra*), 36
Indigenous healing practices, 26, 153
Individualism, xii, 23, 152, 153–54
Industrialization, 40, 67
Industrial Revolution, 85
Inequities in current American healthcare, xii, xxv, 1–2, 149–150. *See also* Marginalized populations; Social stratification
Infant feeding/formula, 64
Infant mortality, 28–29
Infectious disease, 39–40, 42, 74; agents of, 84; epidemic fevers, 89; metaphors, 76–77; parasites, 86–87; pathogens, 86; theories of, 18; in urban areas, 90–91. *See also* Epidemics; Pandemics
Institutions: archaeological approaches to, 96–97; mechanism of control, 97
Intersectional approaches, 6–7, 27, 29, 38, 63, 98, 115, 134–35, 154–55
Irish Americans, 32, 33–34, 42, 54, 146; botanical medicine, 110–111
Iroquois people, 35

Jacksonian-era democratic ideals, 42–43
Jefferson, Thomas, 36
Johnson, Christopher, 38
Johnston, Robert D., 44

Keeping Fit to Fight (Army Surgeon General), 119–20
Kiss, Max, 132
Knights of Columbus, 118

Knoxit Injections, 131–32, *133,* 139
Koch, Robert, 18, 102

Laënnec, René, 19
Larkspur Lotion, 132, *133,* 139
Larsen, Clark Spencer, 64
Late Woodland period (AD 900–1607), 36
Lee, Lori A., 67–68
Leonard Medical School, 25
Letterman, Jonathan, 125
Letterman Hospital, 125, 138
Linn, Meredith B., 42, 54, 110–11, 146
Lister, Joseph, 18
Lobelia siphilitica (blue lobelia), 35
Loren, Diana DiPaolo, 39–40
Lowell Boardinghouse, Massachusetts, 66–67
Lupton, Deborah, 79
Lydia Pinkham's Vegetable Compound, 43, *62,* 62–63

Magdalen Society of Philadelphia, 97
Magnetic and Cold Water Guide, 41
Malaria, 85
Managed care programs, 69
Mapping techniques, public health, 93
Marcus Aurelius, 16
Marginalized populations, xiii, 15, 84. *See also* Social stratification
Mbembe, Achille, 2
McClintock, Anne, 136
McGuire, Randall H., 70–71
McGulpin Point, 149
Medical archaeology, xiii–xiv, 147, 148, 149–57. *See also* Bioarchaeology; Historical archaeology
Medical College of Georgia, 21
Medical education. *See* Physicians
"Medicalization," 59–61; "disease mongering," 65; and gender-based frameworks, 61–66
Medical manuals, 56
Medicine. *See* Biomedicine (orthodox medicine); CAM (complementary and alternative medicine)
Menstrual products, 64–65
Mental illness, 97–98
Miasmic theories of contagion, 92
Midwifery, 23, 29–30. *See also* Childbirth

Military citizenship, 113–14
Military Hygiene for the Military Services, 136
Mineral water, 54–55
Mitchell, Mary, 84
Mohawk people, 36
Mol, Annemarie, 143, 156
Moroline, 53
Morrogh, Clifford, 20, 41
Mortality/morbidity rates, 83–84
Mott, Joseph, 118
Mount Pleasant Plains Cemetery, 30–31
Mrozowski, Stephen A., 37
Mullins, Paul R., 50

Nassaney, Josephine, xii–xiii
Native Americans, 36, 81–83; botanical knowledge, 14; clothing, 82–83; ethnomedical traditions, 35
Nature: healing powers of, 40; metaphysical concept, 40–41
"Necropolitics," 2
New Brunswick, New Jersey, 20, 145
Nichols, Mary Gove, 28
Nickerson, William, 130
"Noncompliance," concept of, 11, 26, 110, 142–43
Nosologies, 18
Novak, Shannon A., 91
Novas, Carlos, 104, 110, 116
Nutrition, 67

Oakley Plantation, Louisiana, 53
Obesity and weight loss, 116
"Off-label" medicine use, 53, 129
Orser, Charles E., 4, 5
Osteopathy, 24
OTC drugs, 138–39. *See also* Drugs; Patent medicine

Paleoenvironmental perspectives, 86–87
Paleoepidemiology, 75, 83–86
Paleopathology, 75
Pandemics, 84. *See also* COVID-19 pandemic; Epidemics
Parasitology, 86–87
Pasteur, Louis, 18
"Past-forwarding," 111

Patent medicine, 51; advertising, 57, 59–61; contrasted with proprietary medicine, 51; criticized by AMA, 57; gender issues, 61–66; history of, 52–53; and "medicalization," 59–61; "off-label" uses, 53, 129; packaging, 72. *See also* Drugs
Patients: patient-led care, 70; patients' rights activists, 51; patients contrasted with consumers, 69–70; resistance to dominant health ideals, 66–69
Patterson, New York, 110
Percussion technologies, 19
Perryman, Lucretia, 30
Personal hygiene, 129–30, *130;* in US Army, 135–37
Petroleum jelly, 130
Petryna, Adriana, 115–16
Petty, William, 89
Pharmaceuticals. *See* Drugs
Phlebotomy, 17
Physicians: diagnostic process, 18; diagnostic tools, 18–20; medical education, 22–25, 27–28; shortages of, 50; standardization and licensure, 23–24; training of, 18; women, 27–28
Pipe use, 83
Pitcher's Castoria, 64
Plant domestication, 85
Plumbing, indoor, 91–92
Pollution, 40, 67
Poplar Forest plantation, Virginia, xiv–xv, 67–68
Populism, 2, 42
Power: and authority, 95–96; state power, 143; state power and biocitizenship, 113; state power and health, 5–6, 144–49
Presidio, San Francisco: analysis, 134–41; artifacts recovered (2008-2009), 114, 126–28, *131;* background and overview, xvi, 113–15, 141–43; biocitizenship and self-care, 123–34; citizenship and belonging, 115–23; history of, 123–26, *124, 127*
Progressive Era reforms, 9, 40–41, 51, 62, 71, 94, 113–14, 118
Prohibition movement, 121
Proprietary medicine, 51, 152; contrasted with patent medicine, 51

200 · Index

Prosper, Kittie Ann, 29
Public health: ancient systems, 87–88; archaeological approaches, 79–87; biopolitical aspects, 75–76; and historical archaeology, 75; mapping techniques, 93; material culture, 87–94; overview, 74–75, 78–79; paleoenvironmental perspectives, 86–87; social constructivist approaches, 94–98; urban infrastructure, 90–94; workplace health, 87–90. *See also* Tuberculosis
Public vs. private space, 156
Pure Food and Drug Act, 57, 138
Puritan values, 39–40

"Quack" medicine, 24, 145
Quinine, 129

Race and public health, 93–94
Radiation exposure, 115–16
Railroad workers, xiv, 32, 55
Rapp, Rayna, 29
Reconstruction period, 31
Recreational drugs, 132, 134
Reflex hammers, 20
Reproductive health care, 26–30, 61–66. *See also* Childbirth
Rich Neck, Virginia, 36–37
Riede, Felix, 111
Rockefeller Foundation, 44
Röntgen, William Conrad, 19
Rose, Nikolas, 9, 104, 110, 116
Rosenberg, Charles E., 104
Rotman, Deborah L., 34
Royal Derwent Hospital, Tasmania, 135
Rural populations, 26
Ryzewski, Krysta, 68

Sandy Site, Roanoke, Virginia, 36
San Francisco, California: Angel Island, 122; tuberculosis case study, 105–9
Sanitary planning, 86–87
San Jose, California, 98
Sassafras, 36
Scalpels, 16–17
Scientific Revolution, 17
Scott, Alyssa Rose, 107
Scott, James, xiii, 6

Selective Service Act (1917), 117
Self-help/self-care, xiii, xv, 50–56, 115, 141–42; and OTC drugs, 139
Sexual health, 113–14
Sexuality, 97
Shryock, Richard Harrison, 23
Sitz baths, 41
Skeletal lesions, 85; and tuberculosis, 100
Sloan, Earl S., 132
Sloan's Family Liniment, 132
"Slum body" metaphor, 105–6
Smith, James, 132
Smith, Monica L., 73
Smith Brothers Cough Drops, 132
Smoking pipes, 83
Snakeroot, 36
Snow, John, 83, 93
Soap and concepts of cleanliness, 136
Social constructivist approaches, 94–98
"Social hygiene," 113–14, 131–32
Social stratification: AMA and cost-fixing, 25; autopsy vs. dissection, 21–22; and epidemics, 111–12; hydrotherapy, 42; and inequity, 84; reproductive care, 29; and tuberculosis treatment, 106–7; in urban areas, 92
Soda water, 42, 54–55
Sontag, Susan, 76, 99
Sorinsville community, South Bend, Indiana, 33–34
Space, public vs. private, 156
Spanish-American War, 121
Spiritual healing, 39–44
Spring Street Presbyterian Church, New York, 91
Starr, Paul, 16, 44
St. Croix, US Virgin islands, 37–38
Stethoscopes, 19, *19*
Stottman, M. Jay, 92
Sun therapy, 41
Surface-Evans, Sarah, 149
Syphilis, 35

Talbot County Women's Club, Easton, Maryland, 28
Taxonomies of disease, 18
Taylor, Dr. and Elizabeth, 43
Thomson, Samuel, 43

Thomsonian medicine, 35, 41, 43
Tobacco use, 132, 134, 141
Tomes, Nancy, 69
Transcendentalism, 41
Trump, Donald, 2
Tuberculosis, 77–78; bottom-up perspectives, 109–11; diagnosis, 101–5; etiologies and symptoms, 99–101; overview, 98–99; as public health concern, 102–4; romanticization of, 102, *103;* sanatoria, 106–9; San Francisco, California case study, 105–9
Tucson, Arizona, 69

Ukraine, 115–16
United States, militarization of culture, 117
United States Pharmacopeia, 57
Urbanization, 67; and industrialization, 54; and infrastructure, 90–94
US Army: alcohol use, 121, 140–41; canteen system, 140; conscription, 117–18; dental care, 137–38; personal hygiene, 122–23, 135–37; pharmaceutical use, 138–40; shadow economies within, 134–35; venereal disease, 119–21. *See also* Presidio, San Francisco

Vaginal douching, 27, 41
Vaseline, 53, 130
Venereal disease, 119–21
Virchow, Rudolf, 18

Wald, Priscilla, 9
Warner-Smith, Alanna L., 94
Water therapy, 41
Wax myrtle (*Myrica* sp.), 36
Wayman African Methodist Episcopal Church, xv, 31
Weimar Joint Sanatorium, 107
Werner, William, 91
Western Washington Hospital for the Insane, 41
White, William A., 58
Wilkie, Laurie, 30, 53
Wine of Cardui, 43, 63
Women: gender roles, 62–63, 107–9; health care, 26–30; reproductive health, 61–66
Women's Christian Temperance Union (WCTU), 121
Women's Medical College, New York, 27
Woodward, Joseph, 18
Workplace health, 87–90
Wurst, LouAnn, 70–71

X-ray machines, 19

Yates-Doerr, Emily, 12
Young Men's Christian Association, 118

Meredith Reifschneider is associate professor of anthropology at San Francisco State University.

The American Experience in Archaeological Perspective

Michael S. Nassaney, Founding Editor

Krysta Ryzewski, Coeditor

The American Experience in Archaeological Perspective series was established by the University Press of Florida and founding editor Michael S. Nassaney in 2004. This prestigious historical archaeology series focuses attention on a range of significant themes in the development of the modern world from an Americanist perspective. Each volume explores an event, process, setting, institution, or geographic region that played a formative role in the making of the United States of America as a political, social, and cultural entity. These comprehensive overviews underscore the theoretical, methodological, and substantive contributions that archaeology has made to the study of American history and culture. Rather than subscribing to American exceptionalism, the authors aim to illuminate the distinctive character of the American experience in time and space. While these studies focus on historical archaeology in the United States, they are also broadly applicable to historical and anthropological inquiries in other parts of the world. To date the series has produced more than two dozen titles. Prospective authors are encouraged to contact the Series Editors to learn more.

The Archaeology of Collective Action, by Dean J. Saitta (2007)

The Archaeology of Institutional Confinement, by Eleanor Conlin Casella (2007)

The Archaeology of Race and Racialization in Historic America, by Charles E. Orser Jr. (2007)

The Archaeology of North American Farmsteads, by Mark D. Groover (2008)

The Archaeology of Alcohol and Drinking, by Frederick H. Smith (2008)

The Archaeology of American Labor and Working-Class Life, by Paul A. Shackel (2009; first paperback edition, 2011)

The Archaeology of Clothing and Bodily Adornment in Colonial America, by Diana DiPaolo Loren (2010; first paperback edition, 2011)

The Archaeology of American Capitalism, by Christopher N. Matthews (2010; first paperback edition, 2012)

The Archaeology of Forts and Battlefields, by David R. Starbuck (2011; first paperback edition, 2012)

The Archaeology of Consumer Culture, by Paul R. Mullins (2011; first paperback edition, 2012)

The Archaeology of Antislavery Resistance, by Terrance M. Weik (2012; first paperback edition, 2013)

The Archaeology of Citizenship, by Stacey Lynn Camp (2013; first paperback edition, 2019)

The Archaeology of American Cities, by Nan A. Rothschild and Diana diZerega Wall (2014; first paperback edition, 2015)

The Archaeology of American Cemeteries and Gravemarkers, by Sherene Baugher and Richard F. Veit (2014; first paperback edition, 2015)

The Archaeology of Smoking and Tobacco, by Georgia L. Fox (2015; first paperback edition, 2016)

The Archaeology of Gender in Historic America, by Deborah L. Rotman (2015; first paperback edition, 2018)

The Archaeology of the North American Fur Trade, by Michael S. Nassaney (2015; first paperback edition, 2017)

The Archaeology of the Cold War, by Todd A. Hanson (2016; first paperback edition, 2019)

The Archaeology of American Mining, by Paul J. White (2017; first paperback edition, 2020)

The Archaeology of Utopian and Intentional Communities, by Stacy C. Kozakavich (2017; first paperback edition, 2023)

The Archaeology of American Childhood and Adolescence, by Jane Eva Baxter (2019)

The Archaeology of Northern Slavery and Freedom, by James A. Delle (2019)

The Archaeology of Prostitution and Clandestine Pursuits, by Rebecca Yamin and Donna J. Seifert (2019; first paperback edition, 2023)

The Archaeology of Southeastern Native American Landscapes of the Colonial Era, by Charles R. Cobb (2019)

The Archaeology of the Logging Industry, by John G. Franzen (2020)

The Archaeology of Craft and Industry, by Christopher C. Fennell (2021)

The Archaeology of the Homed and the Unhomed, by Daniel O. Sayers (2023)

The Archaeology of Contemporary America, by William R. Caraher (2024)

The Historical Archaeology of the Pacific Northwest, by Douglas C. Wilson (2024)

The Archaeology of American Medicine and Healthcare, by Meredith Reifschneider (2025)

Printed in the United States
by Baker & Taylor Publisher Services